DOCTORS' MARRIAGES

A Look at the Problems
and Their Solutions

SECOND EDITION

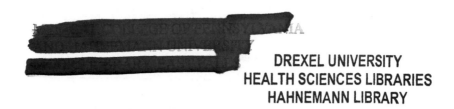

DOCTORS' MARRIAGES

A Look at the Problems and Their Solutions

SECOND EDITION

Michael F. Myers, M.D.

*St. Paul's Hospital
and University of British Columbia
Vancouver, British Columbia, Canada*

With a Foreword by

Carol C. Nadelson, M.D.

PLENUM MEDICAL BOOK COMPANY
NEW YORK AND LONDON

Library of Congress Cataloging-in-Publication Data

yers, Michael F.
   Doctors' marriages : a look at the problems and their solutions /
Michael F. Myers ; with a foreword by Carol C. Nadelson. -- 2nd ed.
      p.   cm.
   Includes bibliographical references and index.
   ISBN 0-306-44618-9
   1. Physicians--Family relationships. 2. Medical students--Family
relationships. 3. Marital psychotherapy--Case studies.   I. Title.
R707.2.M94 1994
610.69'6--dc20   94-100
                                                                 CIP

ISBN 0-306-44618-9

© 1994, 1988 Plenum Publishing Corporation
233 Spring Street, New York, N.Y. 10013-1578

Plenum Medical Book Company is an imprint of Plenum Publishing Corporation

Printed in the United States of America

For my mother and late father,
who share this day

And for Joice, who made this day possible

FOREWORD

A book entitled *Doctors' Marriages* implies that doctors' marriages are special or different from marriages of other people. Why a book, especially a second edition, on this topic?

The profusion of literature about doctors' marriages sustains a conviction that there is a substantial degree of marital dysfunction and conflict among doctors. This is often connected to beliefs that the personality attributes of physicians lead to problems with intimacy, and that the stresses of medical practice, coupled with rigid, compulsive personality styles, contribute to the higher incidence of marital problems, as well as psychopathology, in physicians. While one can wonder at the reasons for the intense interest, and for the perpetuation of these assumptions, a close look at the data fails to substantiate their validity. Instead, one finds a more optimistic picture of satisfaction and fulfillment in physician marriages.

Lewis et al.[1] note that it is difficult to reconcile this positive view with evidence that one out of four physician–spouse couples reports participation in marital or family therapy. Difficult, that is, unless one acknowledges that seeking therapy does not necessarily imply severe dysfunction, but may instead represent a search for better adaptation and happiness. Alternatively, the discrepancies between assumption and reality may come from the fact that we are dealing with different samples; those who are the objects of clinical reports and those responding to questionnaires may not be the same people who are seeking therapy.

Nevertheless, the realities of contemporary life are stressful for all of us, and physicians are no exception. The results of our complex and conflicted lives can be seen in many areas, including the escalating rates of family violence and divorce. Although marriages last the same length of time as they did a century ago, divorce rather than death more often ends them now. Reconfigurations of families often occur in an acrimonious context and families may be drawn into intense loyalty conflicts and rancorous altercations, which sometimes lead to violence, well in advance of divorce itself. There are often no good solutions, only acceptable ones, and all family members bear the burden.

Among the changes that have been blamed for family strife is the "disintegration" of the "traditional" family. That is, the family with two parents, one working at home, caring for children and other family members, and one working outside the home. This description now fits less than 10% of American families. Neither the cause nor the effect of family disruption is clear, but physicians and their families are also experiencing this "disintegration."

We no longer encounter many one-career, two-person partnerships, with hard-working physician-husbands and self-sacrificing, stay-at-home wives. Instead, we see dual-career couples with relationships flexible enough to answer the needs and constraints of both partners, while allowing priority setting and decision making to occur without a "wife at home." The nature of physicians' relationships, commitments, and marriages has continued to change, and the kinds of partnerships that Dr. Myers describes bear little likeness to the "traditional" model of the medical marriage. Today, most physicians, especially women physicians, are in dual-career marriages.

In this book, Dr. Myers has succeeded in presenting an insightful description and providing a rich clinical matrix that enlivens it. He has allowed us to see the skill and sensitivity that he brings to his work with a diversity of physicians and medical students, presenting the array of problems, concerns, and symptoms with which his patients deal. He has also brought us into the world of today's and tomorrow's physicians by taking account of the changing world of medicine and the increasing complexity and differing stresses of physicians' lives. He has defined marriage in broader terms to include a range of committed relationships. In *Doctors' Marriages*, Dr. Myers speaks eloquently, and more broadly, of the turmoil in many marriages, touching a wider audience than doctors.

Carol C. Nadelson, M.D.

Past President
American Psychiatric Association
Washington, D.C. and
Professor of Psychiatry
Tufts Medical School
Boston, Massachusetts

REFERENCE

1. J. M. Lewis, F. D. Barnhart, E. P. Nace, D. I. Carson, and B. L. Howard, "Marital Satisfaction in the Lives of Physicians," *Bulletin of the Menninger Clinic* 57(4, 1993), 458–465.

INTRODUCTION

Although I did not realize it at the time, I began this book on doctors and their marriages during my childhood. Neither of my parents was a physician, nor do I come from medical ancestry. My father was a lawyer; my mother was a secretary who, like most women of her day, became a full-time homemaker and mother after marriage. Theirs was a typical male professional's marriage of the 1940s and 1950s—my father worked incessantly and was the breadwinner, and my mother did all of the unpaid labor of running the home, raising five children. Despite material comfort, I felt personally and emotionally frustrated within this family matrix, and this frustration became evident as ideas and dreams of my own future began to germinate. I knew I didn't want to be a lawyer! Interestingly, my friends whose fathers were hard-working doctors (and with whom it was a relief to gripe) didn't want to become doctors!

As the son of a dedicated, honest, and striving professional man, I grew up feeling shortchanged of my father's time and companionship. His was a general practice of law, with frequent night and weekend calls—someone on his deathbed wanted to change his will, someone at the city jail needed legal counsel—an endless number of anxious clients who couldn't be accommodated during regular business hours. Although my father was not home most of the time, the constant telephone calls of people trying to reach him made his presence felt. My mother never faltered in her defense of his commitment to work and absence from home. To this day her words echo in my ears: "Your father's work is very important—it's not a nine-to-five job." My friends whose fathers were physicians heard similar statements from their mothers. We agreed on two points: None of us took any solace in our mothers' attempts to appease us, and we all felt guilty for complaining and feeling sorry for ourselves.

When I decided to become a doctor, I vowed to myself that I would do it differently; I would strike a balance between my work and my family. How soon I learned that despite one's best intentions, it is no simple matter to get away from the hospital or office at a reasonable hour with a sense of certainty that one's work is done for the day. I married early in my residency; my wife and I began a family toward the end of those training years. I found it a continuous struggle to meet the needs of my patients, the medical students I was teaching, my wife, and my young daughter—plus prepare for fellowship (i.e., board) examinations.

My first exposure to psychiatric distress in the medical profession had occurred much earlier, when one of my roommates in medical school committed suicide. We were both first-year medical students. Although his tragic death was not felt to be related to academic or social stress at medical school, it was impossible not to be guiltily introspective. I will never forget standing before my class the following day and announcing that my roommate had died. I remember my trembling legs and quivering voice and the ashen faces of my classmates. Little more was said about the suicide; I suspect that most of us went underground with our feelings and fears as we threw ourselves into anatomy, biochemistry, and other courses.

While a resident in psychiatry, I gained my earliest experience with patients who were doctors, their spouses (usually wives in those days), and their children. Doctor-patients and their families always make residents nervous, and I was no exception. I experienced a sense of naked visibility and all the other insecurities of being a trainee, yet at the same time I always felt touched by the respect I was accorded and the gratitude paid to me for my efforts. Their attitudes toward me sparked and nurtured the intense curiosity and concern I felt for these doctors and their families whose lives, at least for that moment, were not going well. Whatever the diagnosis, from the most damaging to the most benign, I was fascinated by its dynamic interplay with the profession of medicine. Who became doctors and why? What vulnerabilities do people who study medicine bring with them? Does the practice of medicine make doctors ill? Can anything be done preventively? These were all questions that excited the curiosity of the scientist in me, but simultaneously frightened the ordinary human in me. They threatened my personal and professional equilibrium, for after all I was a physician, too. As I listened to the stories of a middle-aged ophthalmologist describing his depressive symptoms, a doctor's wife struggling with alcoholism, or a doctor's son coming off drugs, my thoughts raced ahead. Is this me in fifteen years? My wife? My son?

Once I completed my residency and opened a private practice I began to see another spectrum of physician ailments—their marital problems.

Not only was I unprepared for the number of doctors interested in marital help, but I felt ill equipped to treat them. Most residency training programs do not offer a lot of supervised experience in marital therapy; those that do may not have many distressed couples who are doctors referred. As is the case with many aspects of medicine, experience is the best teacher, and that experience (coupled with continuing medical education courses and the wisdom of senior consultants) has stimulated and fostered my continued professional interest in doctors and their marriages.

This book is the product of my work. The "data base" that forms its substance includes the more than 130 medical student or physician couples that I have treated over fifteen years of clinical practice. An additional seventy-five medical students and physicians have been treated individually for relationship concerns that include separation and adjustment to divorce. Most of these individuals were treated in my private practice, but a few have been treated in my supervisory work with medical students and psychiatric residents in a teaching setting. Although most couples were married, a few couples (apart from gay male and lesbian couples) were cohabiting for a year or more before seeking help.

My purpose in writing this book transcends the detached documentation of the common marital problems of medical students and physicians or the perspective of one clinician toward the eradication of these problems. I have written from a position of uneasiness—an uneasiness about the present state of medicine in North America and about the difficulty many medical students and doctors are having with their marriages. We are living and working in an era of extremely high marital breakdown with only minimal letup in sight, and the psychological impact for all family members is serious. I hope that this book will be of help, both preventively and therapeutically, to the interested reader—particularly medical students and doctors, their spouses and partners, and their age-appropriate children. I also hope that it will attract therapists to this subject and offer new knowledge to those therapists already working with physicians and their families.

I have organized this book in chapters beginning with medical student marriages, then resident physician marriages, male physician marriages, and so forth. This division of subject was somewhat arbitrarily chosen for clarity and for progression through the marital life cycle. However, there is overlap from one chapter to the next; to avoid being redundant I have tried to cover certain themes more thoroughly in one place than another. For example, if you are a doctor married to another doctor, you will be interested in the chapters on male physician marriages and female physician marriages. If you are a resident and your spouse is a medical student, you will be interested in the chapters on resident physician and medical student marriages. The section on treatment, deliberately set out in the form of questions and answers, is straightforward and should be of practical help.

My orientation throughout this book is a biopsychosocial one, a synthesis of the biological, psychological, and social determinants of illness and treatment. Although this work is about doctors and their marriages, it is much more than a checklist of complaints and simple suggestions. I am a physician who treats other physicians. I approach the troubled marriages of doctors with a "physicianly" vision, and I try my best to appreciate and understand the richness and complexity of the context in which doctors live their marriages. This scope permeates each chapter, and I hope it will be satisfying and enlightening to the reader.

Finally, I have used numerous case examples to illustrate and highlight specific problems and treatment situations. These are composites, usually, of many cases with similar themes and underlying dynamics. They have been significantly altered and heavily disguised to protect the identities of all my patients and to preserve confidentiality.

Michael F. Myers, M.D.

Vancouver, British Columbia

INTRODUCTION
TO THE SECOND EDITION

I have made significant changes and additions to this second edition of *Doctors' Marriages*. My "data base" has increased substantially since 1988—to more than five hundred medical students and physicians whom I have treated over the past twenty years. This increased experience has both yielded new findings (which are included here) and confirmed observations made earlier.

The basic organization of the book remains unchanged. I have, however, reviewed each chapter, deleting inaccuracies, rewriting passages that were vague or confusing, and highlighting findings and comments that are especially true today. For several chapters I have added more references—for readers who wish to explore a subject more thoroughly and to note that there is some, or substantial, research in certain dimensions of physician health.

I have incorporated into the text several more case vignettes than appeared in the first edition of *Doctors' Marriages*. Many readers find it helpful to read examples of the types of problems, conflicts, approaches, and outcomes that I describe in the book. As a psychiatrist, I find it a privilege to become a part of the privacy and intensity of my patients' lives. I welcome this opportunity to share this gift, respecting appropriate safeguards, with my readers; my patients' stories are a mirror for many of us and diminish the fear and aloneness that are so common in physicians facing their own personal struggles.

I have combined into one the two chapters on medical student and resident physician marriages. This large chapter now describes common problems that occur in married trainees whether they are undergraduate or postgraduate students. I have described marital issues that are unique to medical students and to residents separately late in the chapter.

This edition includes an entire chapter on older physicians and their marriages. This is a reflection of a clinical change in my practice:

I am seeing a larger number of older physician couples in my work, and changing demography. We are all living longer; it is only natural that problems will occur during this phase of the life cycle.

Substantive changes in content reflect changes in North American society over the past five years, especially socioeconomic, political, and multicultural waves that influence the profession of medicine and the lives of its practitioners. I have added sections on medical student abuse, residents' economic strain, demoralization and depression in physicians, malpractice litigation, sexual abuse, infertility, HIV and AIDS in gay and married bisexual physicians, doctor–patient boundary violations and other ethical breaches, and stressors for international medical graduates. Where appropriate, I have added clinical vignettes to illustrate particular themes or issues in doctors' lives. The chapter on treatment is largely unchanged—reviewers have found this section to be comprehensive, clear, and of much practical help to the reader.

The most common and consistent piece of direct feedback that I have received from individuals who have read *Doctors' Marriages* is this (or some variant): "Your book gave me permission to go get help for my problems." This is extremely gratifying for me and satisfies my main purpose in writing the book. As I stated back in 1988, "I have written from a position of uneasiness—an uneasiness about the present state of medicine in North America and an uneasiness about the difficulty many medical students and doctors are having with their marriages." I continue to feel uneasy, and this state is what drives me, along with the passion of an old Talmudic saying: "It is not up to you to finish the work, but neither are you free not to take it up."

Once again, any new case examples in this edition are deliberately fictionalized to ensure the privacy and confidentiality of my patients.

Michael F. Myers, M.D.

Vancouver, British Columbia

ACKNOWLEDGMENTS

While attending the 1977 meeting of the American Society for Adolescent Psychiatry in Brazil, I had the good fortune to meet Dr. Margaret Mead and share several hours of conversation with her. We talked about many areas in which psychiatry and anthropology interface, but I remember specifically how much she challenged me to trust and believe in my evolving ideas about the professional socialization of medical students. Women were just beginning to enter medical school in increasing numbers, and I was interested in the sex-role differences in their approach to their education, their patients, and their marriages. Margaret Mead was more than engaging on this matter—she was galvanizing! As was her way, this woman of stature spoke to me in sensible, pragmatic, and dogmatic terms. I came away with many suggestions and a renewed spirit. I know that her inspiration and the memories of that serendipitous encounter have been tremendously sustaining. I have gone on to refine my hunches and ideas, to sharpen the focus, to write, and to speak out on this subject. For the encouragement to do this I am indebted to her. I also credit her with much of my fortitude and tenacity in writing this book.

The late Dr. Nancy Roeske, a professor of psychiatry at the Indiana University School of Medicine, was a friend and mentor to me. She was a noted and highly respected American psychiatrist whose untimely death in 1986 interrupted a brilliant career as a superb teacher, researcher, and clinician. She wrote widely on many subjects—the role conflicts of women in medicine, stress and the physician, teaching methodology, the impact of a handicapped child on the family, the psychological aspects of hysterectomy—and we had many professional and personal interests in common. She was very excited about my desire to write a book on doctors and their marriages and volunteered to review early drafts. I have incorporated Nancy's support of this book by rereading several times one of her last and most autobiographical published papers, "Life Stories as Careers—Careers as Life Stories."[1] It is so relevant to my theme and purpose here, and very comforting.

Dr. Carol Nadelson, a professor and vice chairperson for academic affairs in the Department of Psychiatry at Tufts University School of Medicine in Boston, has also been a friend and mentor to me. One of her many interests and areas of expertise is marital and sex therapy, and her writings on these subjects and on divorce are well respected in American psychiatry. As a former director of medical student education and a current director of postgraduate education, she has long been interested in the marriages of medical students and residents and the delicate balance of personal and professional lives. She and her husband (Dr. Ted Nadelson, psychiatrist-in-chief at Boston Veterans Administration Medical Center) have written extensively on dual-career marriages. These two very dynamic and prolific people are an inspiration to many psychiatrists in North America. I am grateful for their support and belief in this work.

I cannot begin to name all of the many colleagues and professional acquaintances who have given their encouragement and endorsement throughout the writing of this book. I thank all of them for their nods, their smiles, and their pats on the back. They have fortified me. Two must be mentioned by name. Dr. James Miles, a professor and head of the Department of Psychiatry, University of British Columbia, has been a friend and senior colleague. He has nurtured me since I was a junior resident. He never fails to notice and compliment me on some achievement, no matter how small. He is also subspecialized in marital therapy and has much experience in treating doctors' marriages. I am grateful for his tireless and unconditional support. Dr. Ingrid Pacey, psychiatrist colleague and dear personal friend, cannot be thanked enough on these pages. We met during residency and for many years worked together as cotherapists treating couples. My empathic understanding of women in troubled marriages has been heightened by this work, and my ability to apply feminist principles to the assessment and treatment of couples is largely attributable to Ingrid. I am deeply appreciative of her contributions, and I cherish our friendship.

I want to express gratitude to the many medical students, psychiatry residents, and family practice residents who have met with me over the years and talked about their lives, their hopes and dreams and plans for the future, and their frustrations and disillusionments with medical education and training. These "rap sessions" have taught me a lot and increased my sensitivity as a teacher and clinician.

I am fortunate to have many close friends who have been wonderful throughout the writing of this book. Not only have they been curious as to my progress and rallying when I've needed it, but they have remained kindly tight-lipped when I am preoccupied and "tuned out" in their presence.

Janice Stern, senior medical editor at Plenum, has been a beacon since the beginning, when we first discussed my book proposal over the phone. Her enthusiasm for publishing this book, and her faith in its message, has been unwavering. Her editorial eye and suggested revisions have given this work its polish. Likewise, Daniel Spinella, senior production editor, has done a superb job of tightening up the text, examining the prose, and helping me to clarify my thoughts. I thank him for his keen attention to these matters and his easy manner in working with me.

This book, of course, would not have been written were it not for the many medical student and physician patients, and their spouses and partners, who have consulted me over the years. I am thankful to all of them and feel empowered by their faith and trust in me as a therapist. I hope they share my mission in attempting to help others by writing about a subject so dear to almost all doctors. For in essence this is not really "my" book but "our" book as a collective of doctors.

Finally, I come to my wife, Joice, my daughter, Briana, and my son, Zachary. Without them this book wouldn't have been written either, but for different reasons. They enable me to do my daily work and give my life balance. This is their book, too. I thank them for their love, their patience, their joy, and the security of our family life.

REFERENCE

1. Nancy C. A. Roeske, "Life Stories as Careers—Careers as Life Stories," *Perspectives in Biology and Medicine* 28 (Winter 1985), 229–242.

ACKNOWLEDGMENTS
FOR THE SECOND EDITION

Since the publication of *Doctors' Marriages* in 1988, I have been invited to give addresses on medical marriages (or related subjects) by many national, state, and provincial medical or specialty associations throughout North America. I have also given lectures or served as a visiting professor at several medical schools and met with deans, associate deans, and resident and medical student leaders. I cannot acknowledge everyone by name, but I want to thank all of the associations and institutions (and their physician representatives) for their kind invitations, their keen interest in this subject, and their endorsement of my work. I especially want to thank all of the medical students, physicians, and their spouses or partners who have attended these meetings. I have been made wiser by their many questions, comments, self-disclosures, and criticisms. Most important, I have now made contact with many psychiatrists and other professionals in Canada and the United States who are interested in physician health and relationships.

I want to thank Dr. Malkah Notman, acting chairperson of the Department of Psychiatry of the Cambridge Hospital at Harvard Medical School, for her quiet support. Like Dr. Carol Nadelson, she has been a mentor and friend to me. We have worked together on the Committee on Physician Health, Illness and Impairment of the American Psychiatric Association for several years and on workshops at two International Conferences on Physician Health. Her energy is boundless, and her wise and balanced approach to troubled physicians is unique.

Dr. Leah Dickstein, professor in the Department of Psychiatry and Behavioral Sciences and associate dean for faculty and student advocacy at the University of Louisville School of Medicine, has been a cherished friend and catalyst for me. She is known for her passion and commitment to medical student and physician well-being. Together we have taught a course entitled "Treating Medical Students and Physicians" at the annual meeting of the American Psychiatric Association since 1990. We delight in the knowledge that psychiatrists who attend our course return to their home communities to reach out to and be advocates for psychiatrically distressed medical students, physicians, and their families.

My psychiatrist friends and colleagues who worked with me at University Hospital, Shaughnessy Site, of the University of British Columbia, provided great support throughout the writing of these revisions. I am especially grateful to Dr. Sheldon Zipursky, assistant head of the Department of Psychiatry, for his understanding and to Gisela Murray, our secretary, for all of her assistance with my manuscripts.

Mariclaire Cloutier, editor for medical and social sciences at Plenum Publishing Corporation, has been tremendously encouraging about a second edition of *Doctors' Marriages.* I have appreciated our "working lunches" in New York, Washington, and San Francisco because they have stimulated me and enabled me to focus on the task. Thanks also to Eliot Werner, executive editor, who from its birth has never lost interest in *Doctors' Marriages.*

I must again thank my family. My wife, Joice, my daughter, Briana, and my son, Zachary, teach and sustain me. I could not have accomplished a fraction of what I have accomplished since 1988—written this second edition—without their sacrifice, their enduring love, and their quirky senses of humor. I am a very fortunate man!

CONTENTS

DOCTORS' MARRIAGES

A Look at the Problems
and Their Solutions

SECOND EDITION

Chapter One

MEDICAL STUDENT AND RESIDENT PHYSICIAN MARRIAGES

The problems that beset married medical students and residents are more similar than different; hence, their common concerns form the bulk of this chapter. I will discuss problems that are unique to each group at the end of this chapter.

It is generally believed that married medical students are less stressed going through medical school than single students are. Coombs and Fawzy studied sixty-one married and unmarried students through four years of medical school.[1] They found that the stressors of medical school were more severe for the single students. They also found that the stress levels for those students who married during medical school decreased upon marrying. They attribute this difference to the emotional support provided by spouses, all wives in these cases because their subjects were all men. To my knowledge, there has not been a comparable study of married and unmarried women students.

Residents having trouble with their marriages form a very mixed group of people. Some are newly married and are adjusting to that in addition to adjusting to a new city, a new program, and unfamiliar faces. Some who married before or during medical school may be struggling with a new stage of marriage, that is, trying to decide whether or when to have children. Some residents may be pregnant (or have pregnant wives) and find themselves facing heightened and conflicting responsibilities. Others are already parents of young children and are attempting to strike an optimal balance between their work and family lives. Some residents are married to other residents or doctors in practice; they are striving to preserve and protect their time together given their very hectic work weeks. And finally, some are older residents with established marriages who have been in general practice for a while and who are now returning to do a residency. These residents, and their families, are often undergoing major change—psychologically, geographically, and economically.

1

The period of residency training has long been known to be a stressful time in the professional development of physicians.[2-9] There is now considerable literature that documents the effects of rigorous on-call schedules, a high number of hours worked per week, and sleep deprivation on work performance, efficiency, and safety in the clinical setting.[10-14] Studies have shown that 27%–33% of postgraduate year one (PGY–1) house officers develop a clinical depression (including suicidal ideation in 25%) or at least depressive symptoms during their internship year.[15-18]

There have been a few studies of marital functioning during residency. Family practice residents and their spouses rated not having enough time for leisure together as their greatest concern.[19] A questionnaire survey of psychiatric residents by Taintor and associates revealed that 12% of respondents separated or divorced during their residency.[20] Schultz and Russell's study of child psychiatry fellows revealed that trainees with a history of marital difficulties, an emotionally troubled spouse, or actual marital problems during the fellowship were at risk for emotional disturbance and other difficulties.[21] Forty percent of respondents in Landau and associates' study of internal medicine residents and fellows reported marital problems, mostly attributed to training.[22] Husbands of interns and residents in Kelner and Rosenthal's study of ten housestaff complained of fatigue in their partners and lack of time together.[23] And finally, a comparative study of marital adjustment among medical housestaff and attorneys revealed no statistical difference in terms of marital satisfaction in either group.[24] The authors conclude that it is not the work itself that is responsible for marital difficulty but whether or not individuals receive from their spouses emotional support for their careers.

In 1984 Dr. Theresa Isomura (Department of Psychiatry, University Hospital–Shaugnessy Site, Vancouver) and I administered a questionnaire to all women physicians who were enrolled in the various residency programs at the University of British Columbia. Twenty percent of the respondents said that they and their partners had communication difficulties; did not have enough time together; had arguments over finances, work, and sharing of domestic responsibilities; and were concerned about their sexual relationship.[25]

With this as background, what are the problems that commonly confront married resident physicians? I have organized these problems into several categories for purposes of clarity. In reality, many of these concerns blend together and are sometimes an extension or consequence of each other.

TENSION AND ARGUMENTS
BECAUSE OF INSUFFICIENT TIME TOGETHER

All marriages require a certain amount of togetherness for dialogue, problem solving, socialization with others, companionship, shared relaxation, and emotional and sexual intimacy. The actual quantity of time together varies from one couple to the next and also varies within the couple itself throughout the marital life cycle. What is optimal for Couple A may seem stifling for Couple B or conversely quite inadequate for Couple C. Most medical student and resident couples are quite young and in the early years of marriage. Each individual's need for and expectation of affiliation, support, and affection are great.

What happens in so many medical student marriages is that the medical student himself/herself becomes overwhelmed by and submerged in work. In the preclinical years, the student struggles with endless classes, massive amounts of new information, and long evenings of study. In the clinical years, classroom lectures give way to bedside teaching, ward work, and small group seminars. Most students perk up and blossom during these years despite the fact that early morning rounds, long working days, and frequent on-call assignments are the norm.

Gabbard and Menninger describe a psychology of postponement in the medical marriage, which may begin in the medical student years.[26] What happens is that physicians-in-training succumb to the demands of medicine and leave virtually all of the domestic matters (household repairs, yard work, bill paying, cooking, shopping, and so forth) to their spouses with the apologetic promise that they will do their share in the future when they have time. Often this doesn't happen, resentments build, intimacy suffers, and marital discord brews. Medical work and study become so immediate and compelling that the psychology of postponement ultimately proves to be a psychology of avoidance of marital and family matters.

In male resident couples with wives at home with children, a common complaint is about the *quality* of the time spent together. These men defensively count up the number of hours spent at home per week; their wives acknowledge the number of hours, which may be quite substantial, but describe husbands who are exhausted, preoccupied, numb, monosyllabic, irritable, or tyrannical if pushed to engage in domestic or leisure activities. Many residents schedule little or no time with their spouses to go out together as a twosome.

By way of contrast, married women residents are usually aware of not spending enough time with their husbands and children. And they feel terrible about it. They feel torn and guilty and may exhaust themselves trying to function perfectly in all roles. They find it easier and more understandable when their husbands also talk about their not seeing enough of each other. This is a form of acknowledgment of their love for each other. Those male residents who strive for egalitarianism in their marriages also feel very conflicted and guilty if they are not doing their "fair share" at home. Their wives are usually working full-time outside the home and so many of the domestic and childcare responsibilities are divided. They too are prone to exhaustion from trying to fulfill many different roles.

The expressed complaint of not having enough time together warrants deeper analysis, because the obvious solution of prescribing more time together does not always work. One must be aware that for certain individuals having to work very long hours provides a convenient and socially acceptable excuse for not having to be intimately involved with a spouse and children. Being and feeling intimate is frightening and difficult for some doctors.[27] Also, in certain couples with deep-seated and severe marital difficulties, not having much time together provides a compromise solution and may protect the psychological integrity of each partner.

This dynamic was operating in Jim and Sandy's marriage. Jim was a resident in psychiatry, Sandy a resident in ophthalmology. When they came for marital help they both complained that they were so busy that they never got to see each other and so consequently never had time to talk, to go out together, to make love, to see friends together, and so forth. Both longed to complete their present rotations and begin the next ones, which were "slacker." Needless to say when they did move on to new settings, they found themselves still "very, very busy." However, by this time, I knew a lot about each of them and their backgrounds—neither came from families in which people were very affectionate or relaxed with each other—so that I could help them see, in a gentle and careful way, how they were avoiding each other. Also, what was most significant was that each of them had been seriously hurt in a previous relationship (Jim's first wife left him for a classmate in medical school; Sandy's fiancé admitted being gay three months before their wedding), and both feared and dreaded ever being hurt like that again.

FATIGUE AND SLEEP DEPRIVATION

What about fatigue and its impact on marital dynamics? Tiredness and listlessness are common consequences of passive learning (e.g., lectures and prolonged time spent studying). And this is aggravated by physical inactivity. Not finding or making the time for regular exercise is a complaint of many medical students. Add sleep deprivation for those preclinical students who cram for exams and for those senior students who are up half the night when they are on call, and the stage is set for exhaustion. Most students know when they are tired; they can feel it, and they admit to it. Other students deny it. Or minimize it. Or rationalize it. They see fatigue as a weakness, an embarrassment, a failing that is incongruent with their image of a hard-working medical student or a dedicated doctor.

Fatigue tremendously influences marital functioning. The exhausted medical student does not participate as much in the marriage: He or she does not share the domestic chores as much, does not talk as much, does not want to socialize, and either does not feel like making love or does it haphazardly. Most spouses are pretty sympathetic and understanding for a while, especially if the fatigue is phasic and interspersed with periods of normal energy and alertness. But everyone has a limit. The statement of the former wife of a medical student is not uncommon: "I couldn't stand it anymore. We never went anywhere, and when we did, he fell asleep. He used to be a lot of fun at one time. I came to resent him and medicine, and so I left."

Bone weariness and sheer exhaustion are easy to recognize. Most medical students and their spouses have no misunderstandings about this. But milder states are more subtle and ephemeral: some irritability, quietness, preoccupation, procrastination, some increase in alcohol use, less giving of affection, some slowness. These changes are almost always noted by spouses first. And the medical student husband or wife almost always becomes defensive when these changes are pointed out. Why is this? Why is it heard as a criticism or an accusation of weakness? Why is it not heard as an observation of vulnerability to stress and an overture of concern and caring?

As mentioned earlier, the effects of fatigue and sleep deprivation have been studied in the workplace but not in the home. Most spouses of residents are better able to describe the mood and behavioral changes than residents themselves. The need to prove one's ability to endure long hours and sleepless nights has long been entrenched in medical training. It begins in medical school, if not earlier, as students spend hours at classes and endless hours at study. Often it is reinforced by academic faculty and clinical teachers whose expectations of students are excessive and unhealthy. By residency, many young doctors are bragging about the number of hours they have worked without sleep or the number of admissions they have "worked up" overnight. Their fellow residents, patients, and supervisors may be impressed; their spouses and children rarely are.

FINANCIAL WORRIES

Most married medical students are carrying some debt load. The circumstances vary from couple to couple. Some students have loans that began during the undergraduate years, others only since medical school began; some have borrowed from family before marriage, and others only since getting married. In 1991, 78% of U.S. medical graduates were indebted, and their average indebtedness was estimated at $50,384.[28]

Tension and arguments about money are most apt to occur when there has been some recent or unanticipated change in financial equilibrium, for example, sudden unemployment in the wage-earning spouse; unexpected pregnancy; increased expenses for a larger dwelling, tuition, or transportation; and unforeseen negative consequences of speculative investing. Anxiety in one or both partners can rapidly lead to blame and unfair accusations when neither individual is at fault. Unfortunately, many couples do not recognize that the underlying issue is anxiety; they become embroiled in the surface allegations, hostilities, and hurts. This can lead to misunderstandings and distancing.

When Jonathan, a third-year medical student, and Grace, an intensive care unit nurse, came for marital therapy, their chief complaint was "we bicker constantly over money." Grace described Jonathan as completely hopeless with money—she accused him of being careless and self-centered, immature, and shortsighted. She was the one who managed their money, and because Jonathan had run up some debts recently, she now had him on a weekly allowance. Jonathan agreed with what Grace had to say and added that he felt guilty. What he didn't admit was that he felt she was treating him like a child and that he was quietly furious with her.

Their backgrounds were very different, and this helped to explain their present dilemma. As the oldest child in a hardworking and economically disadvantaged immigrant family, Grace had learned responsibility from a very early age. She had worked part-time all through high school and had become financially independent of her parents before studying nursing. By way of contrast, Jonathan was the youngest child of two physicians and although he always had part-time and summer jobs, he had not had to struggle as Grace had. His parents were assisting him with medical school tuition and related expenses.

Grace and Jonathan did well after a few marital therapy sessions. Grace was able to see how her anxiety about money was contributing to her need to control and monitor Jonathan's actions in a way that she herself didn't like. "I don't really want to be your parole officer, Jonathan" were her words. Jonathan was able to see his part in this as well, that is, that he did need to become better informed about their finances, take more responsibility, and work toward greater financial independence from his parents. He also became more in touch with his anger toward Grace, when he felt it, and began to tell her directly rather than withdraw.

What about resident physicians? Many residents have a backlog of educational debts in addition to all the expenses of everyday living—food, rent or mortgage, recreation, and the like. Those residents with children are usually more stressed with regard to their finances. Research has shown that residents with higher levels of medical school indebtedness are more likely to moonlight.[29] Some moonlight to augment their monthly salaries, which paradoxically serves only to heighten the stress in many homes. The stress is heightened for at least two reasons. First, the resident is prone to increasing fatigue caused by moonlighting on top of a regular job and on-call rotation. Second, he or she is away from family even more; this absence can produce feelings of rejection and resentment in those at home. What is gained in one area (monetary acquisition) is lost in another (marital harmony and closeness).

The reader is wise to remember that issues involving money cannot be fully understood out of context. They are best seen as superimposed on unique and very different individuals and couples. For example, economic hardship for a resident from a financially deprived background may be felt and handled very differently than economic hardship for a resident from a wealthy background. Residents and their spouses come from a range of backgrounds, some very happy and secure, others very unhealthy and traumatic. Hence, both their personal vulnerability to marital distress over money matters and their ability to cope with it vary tremendously.

LONELINESS AND ISOLATION
(INCLUDING GEOGRAPHICAL RELOCATION)

A sense of loneliness may develop in spouses of medical students who are studying a lot, or who are preoccupied with anxieties about medical course work. This feeling can also arise if the individuals are not seeing enough of each other due to conflicting schedules, long

working days, and many periods of hospital-based on-call. Both husbands and wives of students are vulnerable, but in my experience it is
more often the wives who are in touch with and verbalize these feelings.
Husbands are more prone to periods of irritability and annoyance about
being alone so much. When they complain, their words may be miscon-
strued as an attempt to control or dominate their medical student wives
rather than an expression of loneliness and a request for time together.
When these feelings are completely unconscious, these husbands are
vulnerable to extramarital affairs.

*Lance was a thirty-two-year-old English professor who had become in-
volved with Sharon, a sessional lecturer in his department at the university.
When his wife, Linda (a fourth-year medical student) found out, their marriage
was thrown into crisis. The two of them talked, and Lance called me requesting
individual therapy "to figure out what I want."*

*Like many people in the midst of an extramarital relationship, Lance was
totally confused. He loved and respected Linda and felt guilty and embarrassed
about his relationship with Sharon. "I'm the last guy who ever thought he'd
cheat on his wife. I've always looked down on guys who do that." His feelings
for Sharon were passionate and overwhelming; he could not imagine giving her
up. Nor could he envision a separation from Linda. Lance and I worked
together in therapy for four months, and a lot happened. He "remembered" that
he had had another brief, two-month affair one year before he met Sharon. He
also told me that he was drinking more over the past two years. He associated
his drinking with going out more on his own. He began to connect these
changes in his behavior with Linda's increased busyness with her work at the
hospital and time away from him. He talked about how lonely he felt in his
marriage. He resented Linda (and medicine) a lot and felt let down by her. Soon
his relationship with Sharon ended. I began to meet once a week with Lance and
Linda together and helped the two of them to begin talking with one another
again. They were now communicating much more honestly and directly. Slowly
they began to trust each other again. They became more intimate than they had
been in years.*

Robinson has described a grieving process in spouses of medical
students who are starting their clinical years.[30] He calls this the "medical student spouse syndrome" and describes three stages—protest, despair, and detachment. Although this process can be seen as resolvable
and adaptive, he urges attention, warning that pathological reactions
such as depression, sexual acting out, and drug abuse can occur.

Some married students make a deliberate effort to keep their personal and married lives separate from medical school and their col-

leagues there. The reasons for this seem to range from the desire to broaden oneself ("Medicine is so limiting. I/we prefer to socialize with people in a variety of occupations and life-styles") to sweeping and judgmental generalizations about medical school classmates ("Who wants to go to a party with a bunch of medical students; they're so immature and socially inept"). I do not take issue with personal preference; however, I do not think it is a good idea to isolate completely from medical classmates, especially other married classmates. I think this isolation can cause and reinforce spousal alienation, which feeds on itself and becomes a vicious cycle. The spouse who initially felt intimidated or rejected by her husband's (or his wife's) classmates now comes to reject them.

I think that sometimes, but certainly not always, these feelings of alienation can be more complicated in spouses who are completely nonmedical, that is, those who are not medical students, doctors, nurses, physiotherapists, and so on. I say this because, despite everyone's good intentions, much of medical student social intercourse does revolve around shoptalk—the never-ending lectures, the "cadaver" stories, a recent fascinating case, or general hospital gossip. Actually, this happens with most professional schools; medical students are not alone in being socially remiss. What is called for is a greater measure of subjective awareness when one is socializing, and a heightened sensitivity and responsiveness to those whose lives and careers are remote from medicine.

What about loneliness in residents and their spouses? Like married students who move to a new city to attend medical school, many newly graduated physicians relocate to begin their residencies. This is generally an exciting time, full of anticipation and challenge. For many, it is their first time living some distance from their families and long-standing friends. In addition to sadness at leaving an established order, it is normal to have some apprehension about what lies ahead.

A sense of being uprooted may be a felt concern for some wives and husbands of residents. The residents themselves are less likely to feel uprooted for two reasons. First, they have the power of having made the decision to move to start the residency (i.e., they initiated the move). Second, they have built-in and substantial institutional supports, such as a secure position, a predictable salary, job structure, the possibility of professional advancement, and the camaraderie of fellow residents. This is not so for many spouses who, often with little help from their physician husbands or wives, have to find housing, survey the job market, find day care facilities, look into schools, and begin to establish a network of friends and acquaintances. Spouses may also have given up a job or interrupted their university education to move with their resident husband or wife. Loneliness and longing for one's family and good friends are common concerns—especially among the wives of male residents.

A lot of couples work through these matters and chalk it up to adjustment. For some, though, these issues are very complicated, especially if they also have some other conflicts they are trying to settle. The spouses feel increasingly unhappy in the host city and may become quite depressed. They may also feel unsupported and rejected by their resident husbands (or wives). With no one to turn to, the feelings of unhappiness and resentment worsen and pile up inside. This can lead to feelings of failure and inadequacy about one's ability to cope with change.

In marriages like this, residents are typically working very hard at the hospital and usually enjoying the learning experience. In contrast, because their spouses are so unhappy, being at home is unpleasant. The residents may suggest ways for their spouses to meet other people and to socialize, but commonly this only leads to more tension, distance, and anger. Making the necessary adjustments is not as simple as that. It is not unusual for both parties to feel guilty—the resident for choosing the particular training site and upsetting the status quo, and the spouse for being so miserable and complaining about everything. A few supportive therapy sessions with a marital therapist can help tremendously with couples in a situational crisis such as this.

SEXUAL COMPLAINTS

I have alluded to changes in sexual relationships in the context of fatigue and what that does to sexuality. There are many other changes in sex that can happen to married medical students and residents and may bring them into therapy. Sometimes a sexual problem is the chief or only complaint; other times it is one of many concerns. In these situations most couples feel that their sexual difficulties are a consequence of the other problems. Usually they are correct.

Joanne, a speech therapist, and her husband, Bill, a first-year medical student, came to see me with the same complaint, "We're not making love like we used to." They told me that they had been married for two years and that their sexual activity had fallen off "dramatically." Before marriage and during the first year, they used to make love two to three times a week. Joanne said they were now having sex about once a month. Bill countered with, "It's more like once every six weeks!" Joanne stated, "I'm the problem. I'm not interested anymore. Bill's always interested no matter what." Bill couldn't make any sense of what was happening to them sexually and couldn't think of any stresses in their marriage or personal lives. Joanne, on the other hand, could, and stated, "Let me tell you what's happened to us over the past year. We moved here last September for Bill to start medical school. That wasn't easy because we've left our good friends [back home] and we really haven't made close friends here yet. . . . My mother died six months ago and although it was a relief, because she had suffered so, it's still a great loss. Bill has been super; I couldn't have made it without him. I'm not happy with my job here and I may have to make a change, which I'm not looking forward to. This worry, plus missing my mom, has made me very uptight. I'm eating more and I've gained fifteen pounds in four months. I hate myself and my body. Bill's out studying at the library every evening during the week; we have supper together, then he goes out. When he comes back at ten-thirty or eleven o'clock I'm exhausted and sleepy; that's when he wants to make love. He feels frisky and I feel frumpy. . . . And finally, Bill's not doing that well. He's failed a couple of his courses and may have to do sups."

My response to Joanne and Bill was simple: "Listening to your story, I'm surprised you two have any sex life at all." With this, the three of us began our work together, which went very well and ended after eight visits.

In the 1990s, disorders of sexual desire are the most common sexual dysfunction in couples seeking professional help. Medical students and residents with distressed marriages are no exception here. But one continues to see and treat other types of sexual disorders as well, such as erective difficulties, orgasmic inhibitions in women, and premature and retarded ejaculation. And most therapists are increasingly sensitive to diagnosing and knowledgeable about treating those adult women and men who were sexually abused as children or sexually assaulted during their early adult years. Medical students, residents, and their spouses constitute some of these patients.

Mike's complaint when he came to see me was "partial impotence." What he meant by this was that he had difficulty keeping an erection long enough to complete intercourse. Although he had had "successful intercourse" on some occasions, most of the time he had difficulty. He told me that he had now become afraid to approach Gail, the woman with whom he lived, and found himself making a lot of excuses so he could avoid lovemaking. Gail urged him to seek professional help. Both Mike and Gail were second-year medical students.

Mike's sexual worries had begun long before he met Gail and could be traced back to his childhood and adolescence. He was an only child whose parents separated after many years of misery and fighting, when he was four-

teen years old. Mike's father, a highly respected surgeon, was a terror at home. He drank a lot and flew into rages during which he became physically and sexually violent toward Mike's mother. Mike frequently intervened and defended his mother, often accepting beatings himself to shield her. Both Mike and his mother lived with this shameful secret in their community to protect the doctor's image. After his parents separated, Mike tried to "become a normal teenager," but he was frustrated and torn because he felt responsible for his mother. She was unhappy and lonely and depended a lot on him for companionship. He felt guilty going out on dates and leaving his mother home alone. She always waited up for him, sometimes half asleep in his bed. On a number of occasions, she made frankly sexual overtures toward him, especially during his last year living at home. When Mike left for college, he felt ashamed and confused about himself and his relationships with women. He contemplated seeing a psychiatrist at the university student health service but couldn't imagine discussing his life with anyone. He feared no one would believe him.

To my knowledge there are no sexual problems or changes in marital sexuality that are unique to medical students and resident physicians. But let me offer some clinical comments based on my work in treating medical students with marital distress and physicians with marital distress who married during medical school or residency. A certain number of these couples were expecting a child at the time of marriage. This in itself is not unusual. But what is distressing for these couples is the degree of upset they continue to feel toward themselves or each other. Because of their advanced knowledge, compared with laypersons, about reproductive physiology and contraceptive methods, they feel foolish, embarrassed, and blameworthy. And sometimes these feelings are inadvertently reinforced by family, faculty, and medical colleagues who are dumbfounded. In these situations, the resourcefulness and tenacity of pregnant and postpartum medical students, residents, and their husbands to adapt to change and forge ahead can be truly remarkable.

For the same reasons, many women students and residents who have had therapeutic abortions are very angry at themselves for becoming pregnant. And I have seen women very angry at themselves because of failed birth control rather than no birth control at all. For most of these women, this very discomfiting time is compounded by their having to go elsewhere (which may be some distance) for the therapeutic abortion in order to escape the scrutiny of medical colleagues and to ensure privacy. I think this self-directed anger and blame is more commonly seen in women medical students and physicians than in other professional women I have treated. This statement, though, is purely impressionistic; I am not aware of comparative studies on this subject.

Sheila, a fourth-year medical student, and her husband, Jack, a journalist, came for marital help for many reasons, sex being only one of their complaints. They were arguing a lot more than usual, literally over anything. Neither wanted to spend any time with the other anymore, and both were spending lots of time with their individual friends. Although they were planning to move in two months for Sheila to begin her internship, Jack was seriously considering staying behind.

I set up individual visits with each of them, and during my visit with Sheila, she told me about a therapeutic abortion she had had two years earlier just before her exams in second-year medicine. Her decision to have the abortion was made carefully and cooperatively with Jack. Both agreed that abortion was the best decision, and she felt that Jack had been sensitive and supportive through the whole experience. Immediately afterward, she threw herself into studying for her exams, then began a busy summer job as a research assistant for one of her professors at the medical school.

By the fall, Sheila found that she was "moody and bitchy . . . I would snap at Jack one minute, and I'd be crying and feeling guilty the next." She began having upsetting dreams about the pregnancy and the therapeutic abortion. She then developed a sleep disturbance—she was afraid to fall asleep. During the day she became preoccupied with something from her past that she had never told Jack. This memory was beginning to bother her for the first time in years. She had been pregnant once before, when she was fourteen years old, and had a therapeutic abortion at that time. She felt horrible keeping this "secret" from Jack, and yet she was scared that he would judge and reject her. She was also frightened that he would be furious because she had not told him about the abortion earlier.

Because I felt Sheila had a low-grade depression that was affecting her marriage, I decided to work with her alone for the brief time before she left to begin interning. As she worked through her feelings of self-blame, loss, anger, and fears of future infertility, she began to feel much better about herself. As she improved, so did the communication in her marriage. I saw her with Jack just before they left the city, and they were happier than they had been in years. Sexually, things were fine.

For some couples there may be long-term consequences of therapeutic abortion if they are not able to talk about their thoughts and feelings with each other. Their marital intimacy and, in particular their sexuality, may be affected.

When I saw Katherine and John they were both residents in internal medicine. Their chief complaint was Katherine's loss of sexual interest. She admitted that this was highly circumscribed and specific only to John. She found herself sexually attracted to other men, masturbated frequently and with pleasure, and had occasional orgasms in dreams. They had no other complaints. I arranged to meet with each of them alone to take a personal and family history. John had no ideas or hunches whatsoever of what might have been contributing to Katherine's changed sexual desire; he did admit, though, that he was more frightened and hurt about it than he was conveying to her. He had gone to the medical library to see if there was anything he could read about becoming "a better lover." Katherine wondered if her altered sexual desire was connected with a therapeutic abortion she had had while the two of them were living together as medical students: "I was devastated when I found out I was pregnant, and so was John. Although we both agreed that I would have an abortion, once we made the decision, John just wasn't there for me. He never mentioned it again and always changed the subject immediately if I brought it up, and I've never pushed. He was raised Roman Catholic and although he doesn't practice it anymore, I can't help but feel that our abortion was hard for him. But I'm only partly sympathetic. I resent him for making this into a dead issue. I don't think it is a dead issue."

Those women and men who are able to work through and come to terms with the range of feelings (anxiety, guilt, anger, sadness, etc.) associated with unplanned pregnancies at marriage and therapeutic abortion are less prone to communication problems and sexual difficulties later in their relationships. Self-contained and reflective individuals will go through this process alone. Most will talk with trusted friends and with each other. Some will talk with therapists. We are living in a time of such divisive rancor and violence over the abortion issue that I fear for young women and men facing the difficult decision of termination of pregnancy. Within our profession, an increasing number of doctors and medical students have become polarized. They are speaking out loudly on this issue. Pregnant medical students and physicians awaiting or having recently had abortions do not know whom to trust. Let us hope that they do not go underground with their feelings.

A Medline literature review of 225 papers on the psychological consequences of abortion concluded that adverse sequelae occur in only a minority of women, and when such symptoms occur, they usually seem to be the continuation of symptoms that occur before the abortion rather than a result of the procedure itself.[31] Many studies report significant positive feelings after abortion and only a small minority that express any degree of regrets. Hence, the "abortion trauma syndrome" is a myth.[32]

Unexpected pregnancy and therapeutic abortion may precipitate a marital crisis. Husbands may have difficulty fully empathizing with their wives' anguish over the decision and the procedure itself. One woman resident stated, "He tries to understand, but he can't—it's not his body, and it's not his career that's on the line." Another woman said, "Is this what's become of me? I've always been so in control of my life—and my body." The more in conflict the woman is about pursuing a residency and *then* having children, the harder it is for her. She feels guilty: "What's happening to me? Where are my values? Is my work this important?" And this guilt will be inadvertently reinforced if her husband is more traditionally oriented than he thought. He will not be very supportive of her decision to abort. He may wonder if she should remain pregnant, try to do it all, or leave the residency. These marriages are really put to the test. I can think of very few times in marriage that require as much mutual love, caring, and understanding.

I want to conclude this section with some examples of common sexual complaints in medical student and resident marriages: decreased frequency of lovemaking associated with busy work and study schedules (i.e., a quantitative change); decreased pleasure and enjoyment in one or both partners when making love (i.e., a simple qualitative change); misunderstandings and a lack of knowledge about each other's sexual interests and arousal patterns; lack of interest in sex in women during the first postpartum year; and sexual withdrawal and distancing in one or both partners due to internal and usually unrecognized conflicts. Again, these are not unique to medical students and residents; they are human concerns. I want the reader to know this. Most marital therapists are adept at diagnosing and treating couples with these concerns.

EXTRAMARITAL SEXUAL INVOLVEMENT

A certain number of medical students and residents come for professional help with a marital crisis precipitated by a recent extramarital relationship. This is a very confusing and painful time for both partners (and often for the third person as well) because there are many questions and few answers. "How did this happen?" "Why am I so in love with the other person?" "Is it possible to love two people at the same time?" "Is my marriage over?" "Have I been unhappy in my marriage and didn't know it?" "Is this just a fling or the real thing?" "Do I have to give her (him) up?" "What about my kids?"

Although there are no ways of predicting which medical student marriages are at risk, let me give some examples from my practice of situations that lead to extramarital crises: the spouse meets and falls in love with someone else because his/her medical student wife/husband is totally absorbed in medical study and work; the medical student or spouse feels misunderstood, unloved, or lonely in the relationship; both the medical student and spouse feel "comfortable," but the relationship lacks depth and intimacy; either the medical student or spouse feels complacent or bored and is looking for some excitement; marital communication is severely blocked; the atmosphere is charged, arguing is frequent, and both begin to avoid each other; a male medical student with a wife and young children at home reacts to the responsibility and "hassle" by seeing someone new; the medical student whose primary problem is within (e.g., depression, alcohol dependence) gets involved in a new relationship that is secondary.

Residents who become extramaritally involved often do so in the workplace. Given the number of hours per week that residents spend in the hospital, this is understandable. At least two factors are in operation: the resident is spending very little time at home, which works against preserving marital intimacy and integrity; and he/she is employed in an atmosphere filled with people who often share a sensitivity and understanding about the stresses of doctors' lives.

One final point. In my work with medical couples, a few are blocked with "unfinished business" about past extramarital activity on either the medical student's or resident's part or the spouse's part. The outside relationship may have ended months or years ago, but the feelings around it have not. I refer to feelings of resentment, betrayal, and hurt. Until these are cleared up (and they can be when the two individuals are mature and courageous enough to talk them through), it is very difficult for complete trust and respect to return.

Pamela was a resident in obstetrics and gynecology; her husband, Owen, was a lawyer. When I asked the two of them in their first visit what their concerns were and how I might be of help, Owen started: "It's very simple. I had an affair a year ago and Pamela's decided she's going to punish me for the rest of my life." Owen went on to say, "She brings it up constantly, at every opportunity she gets. I'm sick of having my nose rubbed in it. It's over. I made a mistake. . . . I hurt her, I know that. I'm sorry. How many times do I have to say it?" Pamela countered, "I don't bring it up constantly. In fact, I hardly ever bring it up, but I want to, I need to. Not to punish you, although at times I wish I could. . . . We need to talk about it. That's why I'm here and why I've brought you here. . . . I don't understand it, why it happened, and how to prevent it from happening again."

Pamela was right! They did need to talk about it because their marriage was in a holding pattern, in limbo; they were coexisting, and both felt miserable. The three of us worked together for several weeks, and in the safety and neutrality of my office they were able to bring out and work through all of their feelings about Owen's affair. They also learned an enormous amount about themselves, not only about how vulnerable they felt in their love for each other but also how strengthened they felt as a couple by coming to terms with this crisis.

PSYCHIATRIC ILLNESS IN THE MEDICAL STUDENT, RESIDENT, OR SPOUSE

Some couples begin to have marital difficulties not as a result of basic communication or sexual issues but as a result of unrecognized or undiagnosed primary psychiatric illness in one or each of the partners. The husband or the wife may be clinically depressed, may suffer from incapacitating anxiety and phobic symptoms, or may be dependent upon alcohol or drugs. These illnesses, in turn, lead to marital symptoms: tension, arguments, sexual disinterest, emotional estrangement, and so forth. This can lead to a worsening of the primary disorder in the afflicted partner, and a circular pattern emerges.

As one can see, this can become very confusing for the partners, each of whom feels increasingly upset and worried. When the individual with the primary problem refuses to accept his or her need for psychiatric help, or refuses to accept help again because of a previous negative psychiatric experience, the situation becomes more complicated. Each partner may feel singled out or blamed, and marital intimacy worsens.

In married medical students, the most common primary illnesses that I have seen presenting as marital problems are depression and substance abuse (especially alcohol). I am using the word *depression* loosely here; there are a wide array of depressed states that include not only the range of diagnoses presented in the *Diagnostic and Statistical Manual of Mental Disorders* (major depression, dysthymic disorder, adjustment disorder with depression, etc.) but also many others: feelings of depression due to the stresses of medical school, feelings of failure associated with doing poorly academically, grief symptoms while coming to terms with the death of a parent, and despondency over one's parents' divorce, for example.[33] These are all personal matters that affect an individual's mood, self-esteem, and sense of control and in turn affect marital dynamics.

Many medical students are frightened or reluctant to reach out for professional help, usually for a host of reasons: a perceived sense of weakness in admitting the need for help, especially in male medical students; denial of the seriousness of their problems; absence of understanding about what might be wrong and that treatment can help; lack of trust that treatment will indeed be confidential and separate from one's academic record; feelings of stigma and shame about having a problem and receiving treatment; a perception that the dean's office is not "psychiatry friendly"; and economic concerns about paying for treatment. Often spouses, who are deeply concerned and worried, feel impotent. The situation may have to reach crisis proportions before help is finally obtained.

Paul, a fourth-year medical student, came to see me after being charged with impaired driving and having his driver's license suspended. His wife, Clare, had been trying unsuccessfully to get him to seek treatment for alcoholism for at least two years. He often drank too much, especially on weekends. During these times he was boisterous, touchy, and sarcastic, not only with Clare but with their friends as well. He had "blackouts" during these episodes, but because he never struck Clare and never drank while on call he considered his drinking "no different than that of any other medical student." His father, one brother, two paternal uncles, and two maternal aunts were severely alcoholic. He dismissed this as "unimportant."

Marital therapy can be an effective route to treatment for primary illness in any person, not just in medical students. For men, especially, it is less threatening and "more normal" to see a psychiatrist for a marital problem than a "psychiatric problem." I find in my work with couples in which there is substance abuse in the man, for example, that he is much more amenable to admitting to the problem and receiving individual help after a few nonthreatening conjoint visits with his wife. And had we not started this way, he may not have ever come for therapy by himself.

Here is an example of a couple who came for help with a marital problem that was the result of illness in one of them:

When I saw Annette and John in my office, Annette did most of the talking despite my efforts to draw John into the interview. Annette complained of communication difficulties throughout their entire relationship. She said, though, that things had worsened over the past three months since John received a mediocre evaluation at the end of his first year of pathology residency. She worried that John didn't love her anymore, because he wasn't making sexual advances any longer and was coming home later and later from work. She thought he might be having an affair; he denied this when she asked him. With all of this, John either laughed nervously or sat quietly in the room, never interrupting or contributing. I asked him about his mood. He said he felt fine.

I suggested individual visits for each of them, as I normally do. In my visit with John I was able to thoroughly assess his mood. Not only was he depressed, he was suicidal. He had recently put his hunting rifle in the trunk of the car "just in case Annette's patience with me wears out." His lack of sexual interest was due to his depressive illness, as was his lateness in coming home from the hospital—he couldn't complete his daily work in the usual number of hours because his concentration was so impaired and he had no energy. I hospitalized John that evening, and he responded very well to an antidepressant medication and supportive psychotherapy. He was discharged after four weeks, and I continued to follow up on him for several months. The three of us met on a couple of occasions, but their marriage was really no longer an issue. Actually, they were communicating quite well together; they both came to appreciate the difference between John's normal quietness and the quietness of his depression.

Let me say a few words about drug and alcohol abuse, which can be a problem for residents. In a study at UCLA, Borenstein diagnosed substance abuse in 15% of sixty male house officers (and 3.4% of twenty-nine female trainees).[34] A further 6.7% of the men abused alcohol. These findings are in accord with several studies of alcohol and drug dependence in physicians.[35,36]

Most married residents with an alcohol or drug problem have marital difficulties as a consequence. In fact, many will not face the problem until their spouses are so upset or demoralized that they threaten divorce unless something is done. I have treated a number of physician couples who present with a communication or sexual problem as the chief complaint when the real issue is a drug or alcohol problem. It may take a series of conjoint visits before they are ready to face their chemical dependency.

It has long been known that impaired physicians deny or minimize that they have a problem with alcohol or self-medication. They may try to treat themselves in an effort to avoid asking for help because they fear losing their license or being expelled from a training program. Many struggle with shame about having a problem in the first place and needing professional assistance. Because chemically dependent physicians have a good prognosis once they are involved in a treatment program, residency directors and institutions need an informational program and a clearly defined, organized process to address the problem of substance abuse in their trainees.[37]

Drug or alcohol abuse that is purely secondary to a primary marital problem is rare. Indeed, some residents increase their use of alcohol or drugs in an attempt to cope with an unhappy or tension-filled marriage, but invariably the problem, or at least the propensity, is present before the marital difficulty. Some will admit to excessive use before marriage; others will have strong genetic loading for alcoholism in their families.

ACADEMIC TROUBLE AND/OR
BEING PLACED ON PROBATION

Doing poorly in medical school, failing a course, or having to repeat a year is a very difficult experience for medical students. Most individuals are not prepared for this type of academic stress because, in general, they have achieved consistently high grades throughout their academic lives. Complex emotions such as disbelief and denial, anguish and sorrow, anger and rage, and embarrassment and shame are not uncommon. Some students are psychologically devastated, suffer a tremendous shock to their self-esteem, and may feel very shaky academically for many months. Some become symptomatic enough to request psychiatric assistance.

This sense of humiliation was illustrated quite graphically in the case of one couple I saw for a marital problem some years ago. Their surface complaints were not out of the ordinary—communication difficulties, frequent arguments, and money worries. My individual interview with Matt, a third-year medical student, was unremarkable. My interview with Ruth, his wife, herself a medical student, was very significant. Her first statement was, "I know Matt didn't tell you that he failed first-year medicine—I didn't expect him to—he won't discuss it with anyone. He hasn't been the same since then and neither have we." She went on to tell me how this blow to Matt's self-worth was at the basis, in her mind, of his hostility and resentment toward her. This was coupled with a sense of shame vis-à-vis his family, which had extensive medical lineage—his paternal grandfather, his father, one brother, and one sister were all doctors. None of them, to the best of Ruth's knowledge, had ever had academic difficulties.

When a married student experiences academic difficulty, this upsets the marital system and affects the spouse. Most wives and husbands are sympathetic and supportive; in well-functioning, happy marriages this is the norm. Other marriages, which are already stressed, may be thrown into crisis or actual disruption by this type of strain. In some of these marriages, the preexisting unhappiness or tension may have contributed to the academic trouble in the first place.

Coming to terms with changing their plans is an additional stress for the spouse of a medical student who fails and has to repeat a year. The spouse may have to work one more year at an unfulfilling job before making a career shift (taking a new job, returning to school, etc.);

postpone starting a family for one more year; endure economic hardship and increasing indebtedness for another year; or delay moving away or returning to family and friends a year later than anticipated. Spouses may feel very bottled up with these feelings of frustration and disappointment; they are loathe to discuss them at home for fear they will make their husbands or wives more upset than they are already. Talking with close friends or family, or a therapist, can be helpful and sustaining until the worst is over.

Let me turn now to residents with difficulties in training, especially probation. Being placed on probation is usually a stressful time for a resident, who wrestles with an inner sense of not quite "measuring up." Usually the probationary period is a finite one, of say six months to a year, and the reasons vary from resident to resident. Some are placed on probation for academic reasons, that is, the resident does not have the knowledge base and clinical ability appropriate to the level of training. Others are on probation because of behavioral reasons; the resident is not conducting himself/herself in a mature and professional manner in clinical work. Some are advised to have a psychiatric assessment and possible treatment if indicated.

Residents on probation may have a host of feelings about it. Some are angry and feel unjustly singled out. They may be petulant and blame the program. Some are embarrassed; they may feel very fearful that their fellow residents will find out about their situation. Most, despite covering up, will feel shaky about their competence in their work and suffer an insult to their self-pride. All will feel under the gun, that their every move is being carefully scrutinized. This feeling, plus the actual enhanced observation by their supervisors, may heighten their anxiety. Some residents can become deeply depressed and suicidal.[38]

Married residents on probation may be touchy and irritable with their spouses, which in turn can spark defensiveness and retaliation in the spouse. Those residents who quite clearly feel sad and down on themselves are more easily supported and reassured; most spouses have no trouble here. But those residents who take minimal or no responsibility for their plight and who are constantly angry, self-righteous, and blaming others have a more difficult time. It is harder for their spouses to be empathic, even when the spouse knows that the surface behavior is just a veneer, a cover for the underlying hurt and humiliation. What is encouraging for residents, their spouses, and training programs is that in at least one speciality (psychiatry), a study of residents on probation tended to show much improvement in the problem area during their remaining training period.[39]

The remainder of this chapter is divided into two large sections:

problems that are more specific to married medical students and those that are more specific to married residents.

PROBLEMS UNIQUE TO MEDICAL STUDENTS

MALE MEDICAL STUDENTS WHOSE WIVES ARE WORKING FULL-TIME

In this situation, there is an enforced financial dependency of the husband on his wife, albeit temporary, until he completes his studies and graduates. Most couples can handle this as a phase of their married lives together. But some cannot, despite enlightened values and espoused ideas of gender equality. These individuals hold more traditional standards than they had realized. He cannot bear to be without an income and feels inadequate; she does not want sole responsibility for financially supporting the two of them and feels resentful. This problem can lead to tension and unhappiness for the couple.

Professional socialization, that is, the personal growth and change that the man experiences as he progresses through medical school and assumes the identity of a physician, may be a source of conflict for the couple. For him, this socialization is exciting and the culmination of many years of hard work and anxious anticipation. But when this change is quite profound or dramatic, it can be unsettling and sometimes frightening. His wife may be jarred by it all and may feel bewildered. The individuals can be strengthened or they may grow apart. They may separate and divorce.

When Sam married Sally, a kindergarten teacher, during the first year of medical school, he was a serious, very conscientious, and industrious student. He admittedly was not very confident academically (he felt "they" made a mistake accepting him into medical school) or socially. He had always been very shy and awkward with peers. Sally, who he met as a sophomore in college, was his first and only girlfriend. She made him feel good. Sam began to change during his clinical years. His grades shot up, and he won a prize in one of his courses after third year. He became and began to feel more popular—he was elected class president. He started working out at a gym and lost weight. He had a brief affair with one of his classmates but put a halt to it quickly. He now found himself seriously questioning whether he still loved Sally and whether to remain married. She also felt confused. She was happy for Sam, for his success and his personal happiness, but she found him distant, preoccupied, self-possessed, and "becoming arrogant." Therapy enabled the two of them to work through and adapt to this change in marital dynamics. In the end, they were

*strengthened and forged a deeper level of intimacy and commitment together.
They did not go on to separate or divorce.*

MALE MEDICAL STUDENTS WHOSE WIVES ARE HOME WITH CHILDREN

These men have usually married before or during the early years of
medical school. Often their wives are pregnant at the time of marriage,
or their children were unplanned and came along quickly after marriage. These couples almost always have financial worries, some of
which are immediate (finding inexpensive or subsidized student housing, budgeting to make ends meet, trying to save money for nights out
or brief vacations, etc.) or long-term (having to pay off debtors at the
end of training dictates and reduces career options). Careful planning
before starting medical school allows some couples to provide their own
financial support, at least in part. Others are wholly dependent on their
respective families, the military, student and government loans, and
part-time employment.

These latter individuals can become very stressed, and marital communication and understanding may break down. Most relationships and
marriages require an optimal period of time for the two parties to get to
know and adapt to each other. When children are born early in the
marriage, this stage in the relationship is bypassed, and deep mutual
understanding and cohesion may be lost. It is overshadowed, quite
legitimately, by the primacy of young children's needs and parental
responsibilities. When I treat couples in this situation, I am struck by
how little they really know each other and how this bilateral lack of
understanding and misunderstanding generates so much of their tension and disappointment.

*When Barbara and Ralph came for marital therapy, they were on the verge
of separating. Life was horrible for each of them, and I imagined it was pretty
horrible for their two young children as well. They could barely sit through the
first visit with me because of so much tension and unhappiness. They interrupted each other constantly, neither listened to the other, both were brimming
with endless anecdotes of how insensitive and unsupportive the other was, and
each was ready to attack. Fortunately, I was able to direct things enough to
learn that their marriage was not unlike a lot of other medical student marriages in which the husband is studying medicine and his wife is home full-time
with young children. I told them that I thought that they were each overstressed
as individuals and therefore in need of some support; they were each expecting
it from the person least able to give it at that moment, that is, from each other.*

I urged them to give me a chance to work with them for a while and postpone separation, if possible, for the time being.

What are some of the issues here? These men may feel over-whelmed and exhausted. They feel the pressures of their medical education and want to do well. This means long days of classes and clinics plus many evenings and parts of weekends for homework and study. The needs of their wives and children compete for their time and attention. All wives have a right to expect a certain amount of companionship, conversation, emotional support, physical affection, and assistance with the children and with the housework. And children have a right to expect guidance, discipline, and play time from their fathers. And these men also have a right to tend to their own needs as well, for example, physical exercise, hobbies and interests, seeing personal friends, or having some time alone. A very tall order indeed!

Their wives are no less stressed. Being home with young children is never easy, even with the supportive friendship of other young women with children, drop-in centers for moms and tots, and available extended family. Young women who are home full-time with children and who are not doing paid work outside the home have the highest rates of depression in North America. These wives of medical students may be carrying far more than their share of the child-rearing and domestic responsibilities of the family and may come to resent their husbands for not assisting them more. They may resent medicine for demanding so much of their husbands. Or they may resent the fact that their husbands are furthering their careers, or growing intellectually, or are at least "out in the world" while they are confined to the home and the world of dirty diapers and unmade beds. In essence, these women are mourning the loss of lives that granted some time for themselves as individuals with some control and autonomy—lives as their own persons and not always as someone's wife or someone's mother.

FEMALE MEDICAL STUDENTS WHOSE HUSBANDS ARE WORKING FULL-TIME

As in the case of the male medical student whose wife is the sole wage earner, there is enforced financial dependence when a woman is in medical school and her husband is working. But unlike the male student, there is less social stigma due to traditional gender customs and expectancies when women are financially supported by men. The revolutionary sex role changes of the past twenty years have modified these societal values somewhat, but not entirely. The stereotypical situation of the intern who leaves his wife "after she put him all through medical school" still causes more outrage in friends and family than the intern who leaves her husband at the same time.

I am not implying that women medical students who are financially dependent on their husbands always feel good about it or have a sense of entitlement as women—quite the opposite, in fact. All look forward to financial independence after graduation. And they are a mixed group. Some have had earlier careers in nursing, physiotherapy, medical research, and so forth and have been completely self-supporting. Some bring savings into the marriage that carry them part way. Some have outside loans and work part-time. Some have never been fully independent financially—they have gone straight from undergraduate training into medical school and have transferred their financial dependency from their families of origin to their husbands.

What are some of the problems that can arise for these women? Creating and maintaining a good level of communication in marriage throughout the years of medical school is absolutely essential. There are many personal and developmental changes that occur in the acquisition of a professional identity. For women this may mean a heightened sense of self-confidence, a greater feeling of intellectual competence, a comfort with making decisions and taking action, and a more secure sense of personal empowerment. These changes affect marital interaction and functioning. Most husbands are excited about and challenged by these changes in their wives. In fact, many of these men, especially physician husbands, have been instrumental in encouraging and shaping their wives' early interest in becoming doctors. They feel stimulated and are supportive. Their own lives may be rapidly changing also (e.g., career progression, promotions, increased professional confidence). When individuals are flexible, mature, and can talk openly, their marriages are bolstered.

Unfortunately, this is not always the case. Some women students enter their senior years or graduate from medical school very unhappy and unfulfilled in their marriages. They feel bored with their husbands, restless, and guilty. They may enter personal therapy or marital therapy at that point. Other women are not bored with their husbands but feel resentful. They find that their husbands give mixed messages. The latter support these changes in their wives intellectually and are seen as being very supportive and egalitarian socially. But they are different at home—undermining, oppositional, petulant, and emotionally withholding. Another group of married women students find they have become lonely in their marriages. They have grown individually, and so have their husbands. But their lives are parallel now, or divergent. They struggle with the decision to remain together or to separate.

DUAL STUDENT MARRIAGES

When both partners are students there is no disparity on financial grounds, because neither is in the paid work force. In general, the couple is being sustained by some savings, loans, and assistance from their extended families. The individual stressors are similar: long days of classes, long nights of study, pressure of exams, and so forth (although there may be differences in how far along they are in their training). Dual student marriages are a mix of pairings, with marriages to other medical students, dental students, law students, nursing students, and other graduate students being the most common.

Let me focus more sharply on dual medical student marriages, as I have had more clinical experience with these couples. With larger numbers of women studying medicine over the past twenty years (the percentage of women enrolled in first-year medical training was 9.1% in 1969; 39.8% in 1991), there has been an unprecedented number of men and women medical students forming relationships and marrying one another.[40] Many of the students are in the same class; many live together during medical school and marry upon graduation or during their residencies.

These couples are subject to the same stresses as other couples in the early years of marriage. Lack of money and differing attitudes toward money management can generate conflict and tension. Emotional immaturity can be a problem when both parties are quite young and have had minimal experience living independently of their parents before marrying. Each may have very unrealistic expectations of the other's availability for sustenance, companionship, sex, problem solving, and so forth. Unrealistic expectations cause disappointment, unhappiness, and bitterness. This is a stage that most couples have to go through. Its passage is much easier for those people who have an outside support group of close friends and family available.

More specifically, dual medical student couples may complain of feeling like they are in a goldfish bowl. There is a sense that the whole class is observing and tracking their every move. How much time are they spending together? Do they look like they had a fight last night? Has Jim been seen in the cafeteria more often lately with Jane (his lab partner) than Karen (his wife)? As they try to protect their privacy and their independence, their actions may be taken to indicate that they are not getting along or that they are being antisocial, especially if they elect not to attend as many social functions with their classmates. An offshoot of this is the reluctance of many of these students to serve as the message carrier or spokesperson for their spouses. One woman student stated it beautifully: "We're just trying to preserve our respective egos—I'm not his clone and he's not mine."

Academic competition can be a problem for dual medical student couples, especially when they are in the same class, but quite frankly, I do not see this often. Sometimes academic competition is positive and enhancing; each partner feels stimulated and pushed to excel by the other. Their feelings of competition are mutually respectful and in good faith. Nonetheless, I have treated medical student couples involved in very destructive and painful academic competition. In the broader context, this rivalry is widespread and extends to many other facets of their relationship. Usually these couples are in serious marital difficulty overall, are literally destroying each other, and are very close to separating.

For some couples, there may be widely divergent academic ability and class standing. She may be getting straight As, while he is struggling with passes and supplemental exams—or vice versa. What is critical here is what all of this means to each of them. When they can openly discuss their grades, and the feelings that are generated by low marks or high marks, and when they can congratulate as well as comfort one another in an atmosphere of trust and caring, there is no problem. But this is not always easy and will lead to tension or distancing when either feels inhibited and not permitted to be frank and open. In addition, many students who are not doing well academically, or whose performance has clearly dropped, are depressed. And this may be misunderstood. They are judged as lazy or not motivated when the problem is that they are not well.

There is one final point about academic competition and marital distress in dual medical student marriages. Sometimes this situation is aided and abetted by insensitive classmates and faculty who themselves are extremely competitive or who have no insight into the downside of competition. Too much of this competitiveness still exists in the teaching of medicine as it has for generations. It is very difficult to change patterns and behaviors that are adaptive, and it is especially difficult to change behaviors that were necessary to get into medical school in the first place! I do not have the answers, but I do know that we can all refrain from comments like, "You better pull up your socks, Diane, or you and Tom will never get matched at the same hospital for your internship" (faculty person to student), or a gender-biased and loaded question like, "What's it like, Frank, being married to such a brainy woman?" (student to student).

OLDER, MARRIED MEDICAL STUDENTS

This category includes both older male and older female medical students who are in their mid- to late thirties. Most have had previous careers, and their final decision to study medicine has been made later. Sometimes this decision is a crystallization of an underlying (childhood) desire to be a doctor that, for multiple psychological and perhaps economic reasons, was not possible before now. Others have become interested in medicine only recently, in part because they have become disillusioned with careers that they have worked at for some time. Some may have been married for several years; others have been married only briefly. Some may have children, infants to teenagers. Some are childless.

What is distinctive about these couples is that the medical student will be adjusting to being a student again. And this takes at least a year, maybe two. For individuals who have been working in another capacity for some years, it is never easy to make this switch, no matter how prepared they are for it. And it means giving up earning wages, not just in terms of dollars and cents, but in terms of independent economic functioning. Those people who have enjoyed quite a lot of freedom and respect in their work, or who have been their own bosses, may have a more difficult time adjusting to the subordinate status of being a student. The more a person is in touch with the ups and downs of this whole transition and can discuss his or her feelings openly with his/her wife or husband, the easier it is to navigate. Mature, flexible, and resourceful spouses can be a blessing.

Another issue for the older married student is a sense of loneliness in the class or isolation from the majority of classmates. Because the individual is at quite a different stage of life, and quite a different stage of marriage in some cases, he or she may have little in common with classmates besides medicine. It the student and spouse are already established in the community and have enough friends and other supports, this is less of a problem. But if the couple has moved to a new city to study medicine, this may be a larger worry. Feeling isolated in medical school can affect one's marriage; needs for friendship and company that are usually met at school or the workplace are not being met. One's spouse may feel overburdened and resentful about that.

Finally, the more in tune that the academic and clinical faculty are with the needs of the older student, the better. When teachers try to respect the diverse psychosocial contexts of their students and are sensitive to age, gender, racial, and ethnic differences, their sensitivity reduces external stress and enhances learning. But when older students are not respected for the breadth of knowledge and experience that they bring with them into medicine, or when they feel talked down to (especially by faculty members younger than themselves) or treated like children, then unhappiness and demoralization ensue. Getting through medical school becomes an ordeal for these students. They become bitter and disgruntled; these attitudes permeate the marriage and can lead to conflict.

WHEN MEDICAL STUDENTS HAVE BEEN ABUSED

Although medical student abuse has been documented for about ten years, there has been remarkably little study of this shameful phenomenon until recently.[41, 42] A total of 500 first-year and fourth-year medical students at the University of Toronto were surveyed and of the 347 respondents, 41% suffered moderate to severe aftereffects of abuse received during medical training.[43] Abuse incidence became progressively higher from the first year to the fourth year of medical school. The researchers noted three types of abuse: verbal abuse (86% by year four), sexual harassment (36% by year four), and physical abuse (18% by year four). Hospital staff physicians were the most frequent source of abuse, followed by residents. Because medical student abuse is somewhat institutionalized and has been happening for decades, many students are not even aware that what they are feeling (i.e., symptoms of posttraumatic stress disorder) is a result of being abused. In a recently reported longitudinal study of the effects of abuse, Richman et al. noted several symptoms and behaviors in students: depression, drinking, leaving medicine, disparaging the profession, ignoring the emotional needs of patients, and repeating the pattern of abuse toward students and others.[44]

Living with abuse as a medical student affects one's marriage in a lot of different ways. Many spouses are outraged and are the ones who first realize that their husband or wife is being abused; hence, they may be instrumental in reporting it and getting something done. Some spouses may not see it at all, however, and either do not believe or otherwise negate what their husband or wife is telling them. In some marriages, there may be displacement from the workplace (i.e., the medical student takes out his or her aggression from abuse at the hospital on the family at home). Some medical students, particularly women students who have been sexually harassed, become demoralized, despondent, and blame themselves. Their husbands may have no idea what is happening and become frustrated, impatient, and condemnatory as marital communication worsens. The charge to medical schools is clear: Deans need to become aware of and sensitive to medical student abuse in their own "homes"; preventive educational programs for faculty (about what constitutes abuse) need to be constructed; sexual harassment committees must be established in all medical schools; and counseling and advocacy services for abused students and their spouses must be available.

WHEN PARENTS INTERFERE IN THE MARRIAGE

If normal familial boundaries between one's marital relationship and one's relationship with parents or parents-in-law do not exist, there may be trouble. What happens is that one's right to privacy and independent living is not acknowledged and protected. And this can create marital conflict, especially when the two individuals do not agree on their perceptions. For example, a woman may find her father-in-law intrusive, but her husband does not see his father's behavior as intrusive at all and defends it as normal interest and caring. He may add or imply that she is being unduly critical, ungrateful, and territorial. She feels attacked, hurt, and unsupported by her husband. He feels torn and conflicted and wonders how he can avoid upsetting two people he loves and cares about.

For married medical students, problems with parents are most apt to occur under certain circumstances: when one lives in the same city as they do; when one of the parents is on his/her own (e.g., widowed or divorced parents whose well-being the son or daughter feels responsible for in many ways); when the parents have minimal or no understanding of the rigors of medical school and complain bitterly that "the kids" do not call or visit often enough; when parents have outdated sex role expectancies of their medical student son or daughter (e.g., one mother bemoaned her daughter's serving fast-food meals to her family the evenings after being on call); and when the medical student couple is almost completely financially dependent on their families. These problems can be very complicated, especially if the couple is living in the parents' home or in very close proximity. The couple cannot help but feel beholden and thereby anxious that they are playing by the parents' rules. And in these families there can be confusing power plays in operation that make it very hard for people to function as adults. Parent–child transactions tend to dominate and lead to acrimony in these situations.

WHEN MEDICAL STUDENTS INTERMARRY

Intermarriage, whether interfaith, interethnic, or interracial, is increasingly common in our pluralistic society and therefore not uncommon in medical students. Egon Mayer, in his book *Love and Tradition: Marriage between Jews and Christians*, describes interfaith marriages as testimonials to a belief in the changeability of culture and society, as well as an ideology of evolution, of rebirth, of boundless human potency for novelty and new beginnings.[45] Indeed, people who intermarry describe the excitement, wonder, challenge, and enrichment of their lives together and the blending of very different backgrounds, customs, and values. But these marriages are not without their share of problems, in addition to the range of problems that beset all couples and are not influenced by race, ethnicity, or religion.

Let me briefly mention some of the more common conflict issues. This is a complex subject, and I do want to alert the reader to problems that can arise. I also want to normalize the conflicts that occur frequently and are transitory. First, there may be an underestimation of the cultural or religious differences between the two individuals. These differences do not seem so great at first but may seem so later or at a time when things are not going well. Each partner may feel that the other is trying to "change" him or her or is expecting the other to adopt his/her attitudes or beliefs more than one can. Each may feel defensive, misunderstood, and frightened. They retreat to feeling that "someone of my own kind" would understand. They may feel they are mourning many cherished values and ideas of their pasts. This is often an isolated feeling.

Second, their families may be having difficulty accepting their relationship; this adds stress to their marriage. Both may feel caught in the middle between the person they have married and their parents and siblings. Sometimes it is only one side of the family struggling with acceptance. This can be more easily understood and predicted the more that all parties come to explore and uncover the unspoken family rules, prohibitions, and generations of tradition. These are not ideas and attitudes that can change overnight. Most families soften with dialogue and passage of time. Some never come to accept the marriage.

Cindy and Charles had been married for six months when they came for marital help because of constant arguing and fighting about Cindy's family. They had lived together for two years before their wedding, which Cindy's parents refused to attend; consequently, they were married in a simple civil ceremony with only a few friends present. Cindy was Asian, Charles Caucasian. Both were graduating in a few months and going away to intern. Charles was bitter and furious at Cindy's parents because they refused to accept him as their son-in-law. He could barely contain the rage, which he also felt guilty about because he knew that Cindy was in the middle. Cindy was quite philo-

sophical; she could empathize with her parents, who were immigrants and had never had to face intermarriage with their other children or within their large extended families. She felt that if she continued to talk with her parents and not reject them, over a period of time they would accept Charles. In fact, she envisioned a "proper wedding" in the future that would be a true celebration of their love and acceptance. This was indeed what happened—two years later.

Third, social stigma and prejudice can add stress to the most loving and harmonious of couples. Its effects are less pervasive for "thick-skinned" individuals and couples but it is never easy, and it is not easy for children. In general, people in medicine tend to be on the liberal, less rigid, and accepting end of the spectrum, but there are many exceptions. And people's attitudes in the workplace, especially in the hospital with its ethos of compassion and care for all, are not necessarily their attitudes in their personal and private lives. I have treated interracial medical student couples who clearly do not feel accepted by their classmates and faculty outside of the medical school and hospital setting.

WHEN FAMILY MEMBERS ARE DOCTORS

A significant percentage of medical students have blood relatives who are physicians. Most often this is one's father, and occasionally one's mother; more and more students have sisters and brothers who are doctors. These relatives are important role models and often were strong identification figures when the student was growing up. In some families the process of identification begins very early, with students reporting their interest in becoming physicians as far back as they can remember. Most physician parents are proud of and excited about their son's or daughter's acceptance into medical school. However, coming from a family of physicians may be a problem for some medical students. They may suffer a "crisis of confidence" or a type of existential career crisis sometime during medical school: Do I really want to be a doctor? In my heart, am I cut out for medicine? Do I truly enjoy it? Have I indeed given this a lot of thought, or am I studying medicine just because my father (or mother, brother, etc.) did? I wonder if I am just looking for acceptance by following in his/her footsteps. For most students, these questions and doubts are quite normal, healthy, and transient; for others, they are quite serious and do point to underlying personal and family conflicts that require exploration and resolution in psychotherapy.

These individuals may have feelings of inadequacy if a physician parent is a highly respected and successful practitioner in the community or a prominent faculty person at the medical school. Or there may be feelings of inferiority if an older brother or sister did better academically, socially, or athletically while attending medical school. These are classic family dynamics in which someone is a "hard act to follow." At the moment this is more commonly a male gender issue, but as larger numbers of physician mothers have daughters in medical school there may be some gender-specific conflicts. For example, a medical student may feel inadequate if she is struggling academically in medical school and her mother was a "gold medalist." Or a medical student may not respect her physician mother for making her own ambitions secondary to her husband's career and assuming primary responsibility for the home and children.

For the married medical student, these intrapsychic and interpersonal difficulties with medical family members may spill over into the marriage. Spouses who do not appreciate these types of issues will not feel very supportive and considerate; their medical student husbands or wives will feel alone and resentful. These feelings will be magnified if the students are financially dependent on the physician parent(s) or if the parents seem to interfere. Some parents who are doctors have very mixed feelings about their son or daughter marrying during medical school in the first place, especially if they themselves waited until they graduated. If the spouse is nonmedical, he or she may feel very intimidated and overpowered by strong bonds and affinity among family members who are doctors. This type of friction is more apt to occur in those families in which the married student is attending medical school in the same community where his/her parent(s) live and practice. It may be very difficult to establish and maintain clear boundaries in one's marriage without the parents feeling hurt or resentful.

One final concern that may affect medical students and their marriages when family members are doctors is the demoralization that is so common in physicians today. A poll taken in 1989 by the Gallup Organization for the American Medical Association found that nearly 40% of all doctors probably or definitely would not go to medical school if they were in college today.[46] Close to two-thirds of physicians surveyed in the Minneapolis–St. Paul area said that they would not want their children to go into medicine.[47] It is quite possible, then, that at least some contemporary married medical students find their physician parent(s) quite unsupportive.

WHEN A PARENT DIES DURING THE MEDICAL SCHOOL YEARS

A certain number of individuals, while in medical school, lose a mother or father to death. Usually the dean's office is informed and the student takes a few days to a week away from classes to attend the funeral and be with family members. Very quickly he or she is back at school and carrying on as before. Classmates vary in their ability to acknowledge the loss, to pay their respects, and to extend themselves in a sympathetic and supportive manner.

Coming to terms with the loss of a parent takes time; normal bereavement has wide parameters of emotional reactivity, coping ability, and duration of upset. Many factors color the grieving process, and some students will have more difficulty than others. I feel that many students do not give themselves an adequate period of time to mourn. Some are not accorded enough time to mourn, or they do not know what to expect. Most of them are young and in their twenties; this is their first major loss, and they are usually losing a parent prematurely as well. These are not individuals in midlife losing a parent in late life. Too many students bury themselves in their schoolwork and studies, which works (but usually only temporarily) to ward off feelings of anxiety, sorrow, anger, and guilt. These may burst forth later or manifest themselves obliquely in behavioral change—absenteeism, academic failure, drug taking, and sexual acting out.

Married students may underestimate how much losing a parent affects them and their spouses. The couple may present marital symptoms (e.g., arguing a lot, avoiding each other, or withdrawing sexually), but the real cause is unresolved grief. I have found this to be more common in the marriages of male medical students than female, and it is their wives who have been worried about their husbands all along. What follows is classic:

"We were fine until a year ago when Bob's father was diagnosed with pancreatic cancer. He was only fifty-two and so healthy. And it all happened so fast; he was dead in three months. Bob says he's fine but he's not. He's touchy, won't talk about it, is very irritable, yells at me one minute and apologizes the next. I yell back just to assert myself. I know he's in pain, but so am I."

Most medical schools do not adequately teach about dying, death, and bereavement, either didactically by lecture or seminar or experientially at the bedside or after patients die. Most commonly, medical students are taught by clinicians whose feelings are pretty much in check as they either attend to very sick patients or counsel newly bereaved families in hospital corridors and waiting rooms. This approach is necessary and adaptive, but I think we can do it better. Medical students need to hear residents and attending staff speak more openly about *their* feelings around death and dying: "I've been practicing medicine for twenty years, and I still find it hard treating patients who are dying," or "This is tough work talking to relatives," or "I hate asking for autopsies, although I know how important they are," or "Since my own mother died, I find that I'm not as afraid of talking to patients who are dying as I used to be; I'm more real now."

With more of this kind of teaching and role modeling, I think that medical students who lose a parent might understand a bit better what to expect. Perhaps they would not feel the need to be quite so stoic, cool, or private. They could allow themselves to experience all of the normal emotions when a loved one dies.

PROBLEMS UNIQUE TO RESIDENTS

ADJUSTMENT TO RESIDENCY TRAINING IN JUNIOR TRAINEES

Some residents struggle with inner conflicts about their chosen specialty. These include self-doubts, lack of professional confidence, an inner sense of disequilibrium, second thoughts about their career choice, and conflicts with authority figures. Conflicts such as these are more apt to contribute to marital tension and estrangement in those residents who tend not to disclose their concerns to their spouses or who tend to play down the magnitude of their internal distress. This stance may be more common in male residents than female residents, but it is not exclusively a male style; I have treated a few women residents who were having major adjustment difficulties and were talking to no one about their distress.

Rob, a second-year resident in internal medicine, called to make an appointment with me and told me over the phone, "My wife says I'm driving her nuts. Unless I get some help, she says she's going to leave me." I met with him, and he described feeling increasingly irritable and "short-fused" for the previous six months. He wasn't sleeping well, and his appetite was off a bit. He also complained of various aches and pains—more headaches than usual, low back pain in the morning, abdominal distress from time to time, and a lot of fatigue after strenuous exercise. His family physician had done a series of lab tests after a complete physical exam and felt he was physically fine but probably working too hard. He told me that his wife couldn't stand hearing about his health concerns, and she was fed up with his outbursts of temper and his criticism of her.

What was revealing in my early work with Rob was how much he hated his job. At first I thought this was because he was depressed, and once his mood lifted he would be fine about it. However, the problem was the other way *around—it was his work that was depressing him. Rob had wanted to be an internist as far back as he could remember. This choice had something to do with his uncle, who was a cardiologist and who was like a surrogate father to him. Rob admired and respected him tremendously. During the first year of his residency, he felt feelings of disillusionment and frustration but dismissed them as "growing pains." They never really went away. He began to resent being on call and preparing cases for grand rounds. He found reading the journals a drag. He reacted to all of this by feeling guilty and depressed. Eventually, he spoke with the program coordinator and took a leave of absence to give himself more time to think about his future. Soon he decided to leave the residency and begin general practice. He and his wife were fine again.*

All new jobs require a period of breaking in and feeling one's way. Residency is no exception, especially if one is not quite certain regarding one's choice of specialty, or if one is entering a residency after a period of years in an established family practice, or doing locum tenums, or doing emergency medicine work. What is essential is that the resident be prepared for this breaking-in period, accept it as being normal, and begin to talk about it.

DEVELOPMENTAL CHANGES IN THE RESIDENT ASSOCIATED WITH SPECIALTY TRAINING

Considerable developmental and maturational changes occur in residents as they progress through their years of residency. These changes include the acquisition of a professional identity, an increased sense of autonomy, and a greater sense of self-esteem. Other developmental and nonvocational tasks include a higher degree of separation and independence from their families of origin, the establishment of a more secure sexual identity, an increasing ability to form and maintain intimate relationships, and early attention to community and social responsibilities.

All of these changes have a marked influence on marital equilibrium. Many residents are acutely aware of the ways in which they are evolving into more mature and secure adults. Some also note the ways in which they are perceiving their spouses differently, particularly toward the end of their training. These perceptions can be upsetting and frightening, throwing residents into periods of doubt and perplexity about their marriages. Comments such as "I'm not sure how much I love her anymore—I'm not the same person she married back in medical school"; "All I want to do is my work—the hospital's my life—I'm totally bored at home"; and "I feel I've outgrown him—I've got nothing to say to him anymore" are illustrative.

Spouses also perceive changes in their resident husbands and wives. And these feelings can be very unsettling because they may signal a marriage in trouble, perhaps in serious trouble. One woman stated, "I don't know if I still love him or not. I know I care about him and his success, but he's so full of himself. Surgery is his life; the children and I are secondary. He says I'm just jealous. Honestly, I'm not." And the husband of an internal medicine resident commented, "I'm very proud of her. She has truly blossomed over the past three years. But I don't think we're going to make it as a couple; I'm much more of an old-fashioned guy than I thought I was."

A theme that runs through these marriages is that the resident alone is making major changes throughout the postgraduate years. This is often a misperception. What tends to be ignored are the different, but no less significant, maturational changes occurring in the spouses. In other words, the problem is not so much that the resident is outgrowing his wife or her husband but that each partner is changing and growing in similar and different ways without adequate understanding, acknowledgment, and dialogue on the matter. When couples can recognize that this is happening and can talk together about it, many of the fears and self-doubts are eased. Their marriage may not be as dismal as they have each thought.

This was the case for Frank and Maxine who came to see me during the last six months of Frank's residency in general surgery. Although Frank had plans to separate and move out within two weeks, he agreed to come with Maxine "for one visit." They were both thirty-two years old. They had been married for nine years, and had children six and four years old. Frank was very clear that his marriage was over. "I don't feel good about this, but I need to be on my own. I've paid my dues. I've been married for almost ten years and it seems like twenty. . . . We've grown apart. Maxine's no fun anymore. . . . There's more to life than young kids and decorating homes. Our friends are just as boring." Maxine, although hurt and furious, had no doubts about her love for Frank. "I can't stop him. He's right, my interests are the home and family. I think he's having an early midlife crisis."

Frank and Maxine did separate but continued to talk to each other fairly regularly in connection with Frank's visits with the children. Maxine came back for a few supportive psychotherapy visits, largely with concerns about the kids and their adjustment to the separation. Nine months later, Frank called asking to see me. He was very different at that visit and had a lot of regrets about leaving the marriage. He told me that he had actually been having an affair for six weeks before he separated but decided not to tell anyone about it. That relationship ended a few weeks after he and Maxine began living apart. Since then he had dated "lots of different women—all knock-outs—but there's something lacking. I can't help missing many of the things I hated about being married—the routine, Maxine's cooking, seeing the kids on a daily basis, even our 'boring' middle-class friends! I never gave Maxine any credit for the way she's grown and changed through our marriage. I just put her down for gaining a few pounds after the kids came along and compared her in my mind with the twenty-one-year-old nurses in the operating room ... nurses who have never even had kids, for God's sake! ... Our sex life may have lost a lot of its spontaneity and electric charge, but it really wasn't that bad."

I suggested to Frank that he begin to talk more openly with Maxine about these feelings and that they begin to "date" each other, if Maxine was interested. She wasn't at first, partly because she was seeing another man, but mainly because she didn't trust Frank's change of heart. They did start going out together a few weeks later, very casually and intermittently. Their time together as a couple, and as a family, slowly increased in comfort and in intimacy, and after seven months they were reconciled.

ANXIETY OVER CERTIFICATION EXAMS

Senior residents may become preoccupied with preparing for specialty certification exams during their final year of residency. This will mean spending increasing amounts of time in individual or group study. For their spouses and children, this results in less time for family activities and responsibilities. Feelings of resentment, varying in intensity, may surface in their husbands and wives; many arguments and misunderstandings may be a direct consequence of this fact.

Residents may also be struggling with two conflicting sentiments, eagerness to be out of training and doubts about being fully competent as specialists. Some will be busy trying to line up practice opportunities, fellowships, or junior academic positions. Those who are obliged to relocate in order to secure a position will have the additional burden of leaving a familiar work setting.

Although these are issues that are common and confront many married residents, they can become overwhelming for couples who are distressed. They are challenges that require a good sense of individual self-worth, flexibility, maturity, and the ability both to communicate clearly one's needs and feelings and to argue constructively. This may be no easy task!

SPOUSAL FEARS OF ABANDONMENT TOWARD THE END OF TRAINING

I find that this concern is more commonly expressed by the wives of male residents, especially those women who are home full-time with young children and who have married before or during medical school. And this is quite understandable, given that these are women who have no paid income for their work at home. Even if they are working part-time, what they earn is only a fraction of their husband's present or future salary. Psychologically, they may also feel they are in a completely different world than their husbands' work world. They are either familiar with statistics on marital breakdown for physicians or are personally acquainted with women whose story has become all too familiar: "He left me right at the end of residency for a younger woman—after I put him through medical school and supported him emotionally all through his training."

Husbands of women residents also have fears of being abandoned, but they are less likely to express these fears directly. Indeed, they may not be consciously felt. What happens is that these husbands may become possessive and jealous regarding their wives' male acquaintances and coworkers. They may go on to develop an excessive need for control in the relationship or become dependent and clinging. Some withdraw into self-protective behavior, as if being left was inevitable.

Let me say a bit more about this. It is a reality that those marriages contracted during the undergraduate years are at risk for marital breakdown during or after residency.[48] The jokes about the frequency of divorce among surgical residents are not funny when one begins to look seriously at the morbidity rates of individuals in divorcing families. Most research has addressed male physician marriages[49-51] and doctors' wives[52-54]; less has been written about female physician marriages[55,56] and doctors' husbands.[57,58] With increasing numbers of women in medicine, spousal fear of abandonment is no longer exclusively a "woman's problem"—an increasing number of husbands struggling with abandonment are seeking help.[59,60]

ROLE STRAIN

Role strain has been defined as "the felt difficulty in fulfilling role obligations"[61] and is a complaint in many resident couples, especially those with children. Tension and arguments erupt over dividing up household chores, marketing, looking after the children, paying bills, visiting extended families, and planning social and recreational events. Role strain is more frequently a complaint for women residents, most of whom either attempt to take on more than their share of domestic responsibilities or are expected to by their husbands. Those marriages with husbands who are truly less traditional (not just apparently so) and who initiate and accept household tasks are less burdened with role strain.

Role strain has long been known to be a problem for women in the professions, and hence its prominence in women residents is not surprising.[62,63] In addition to their clinical and academic responsibilities in the hospital setting, these women not only perform more than their share of homemaking and child care but also organize and manage most of it. These responsibilities often result in feelings of exhaustion, at times resentment, and without exception guilt. One woman's statement says it all: "I'm never guilt free. When I'm home with my daughter, I feel I should be with my patients; when I'm at the hospital on call, I feel I should be with my daughter and my husband; when my mother visits, I feel the house is a mess; when I'm at a movie, I feel I should be studying."[64]

Role strain in male physicians has been studied less.[65,66] Historically, the male physician has been able to devote all or most of his energies to his medical career because he has had a wife at home to do everything else. Today, many male physicians' wives are working outside the home, and the trend is toward an attempted sharing of domestic and child-care responsibilities. Increasingly, men are feeling the tension and exhaustion of competing conflicts between their work, marriage, and children. It seems that all but the most traditional of medical marriages will continue to move in this direction.

WHEN A RESIDENT IS PREGNANT

A study by Sayres and associates found that one in eight married women in Harvard-affiliated programs was pregnant in 1983.[67] Their study also revealed the paucity of formal maternity-leave policies; four-fifths of the programs did not have one. Further, they found that residents rated their pregnancy experience more favorably if the program director was supportive, if pregnancy during training was openly discussed, and if the resident was allowed to resume work part-time for the early weeks after maternity leave. The authors make several suggestions for easing the problem for pregnant trainees and program directors.

Since Sayres and associates' study, the American College of Physicians has issued a position paper on parental leave for residents. This document emphasizes the needs of pregnant trainees and their spouses and provides guidelines to program directors and institutions. Although many more programs have maternity leave policies now than a decade ago, some do not. And many include only maternity provisions, not leaves for fathers or to facilitate adoption.[68]

What are the implications of all of this for married residents and their husbands? First, directors of postgraduate education in medical schools and residency programs in hospitals have to accept that pregnancy in some residents during training is a reality that is here to stay. Second, they have to support residents who become pregnant formally through institutional policy changes regarding implementing and updating maternity leave, coverage, and so forth, and informally through direct acknowledgment, interest, and simply caring about their trainees' personal and family lives. Third, there needs to be strong and repeated recognition of the fact that measures of residents' marital happiness do not exist in a vacuum, that peoples' personal lives are deeply affected by psychosocial stressors in the workplace (and vice versa). There is a direct and interdigitating relationship.

Pregnancy, especially when planned, is an exciting and usually joyous process for the woman and her husband. Yet it can be stressful, less than happy, and associated with marital conflict. Many pregnancies during residency are unplanned (e.g., as a result of inadequate, failed, or no contraception). Some residents inadvertently become pregnant just as they are about to separate from their husbands. Some separate during the pregnancy or the first postpartum year. Some women doctors who come for couple therapy while their children are young trace the origins of their marital difficulty back to the time of their residencies. They recall high stress as they tried to prepare for becoming a mother as well as meet their husbands', patients', and programs' needs.

I am alarmed by what I see happening to the personal and marital lives of many residents who start their families during postgraduate training. I feel that radical changes must occur in the outdated and discriminatory attitudes of some program directors, or, failing that, these individuals must be replaced. Many types of specialty training and specific programs need serious study and revision to accommodate and recruit women applicants who are in their childbearing years. How many more physician divorce casualties do we need in order to make the residency years more humane and respectful of family life?

WHEN A RESIDENT IS AN INTERNATIONAL MEDICAL GRADUATE (IMG)

International medical graduates (IMGs) are subject to an enormous number of stresses that may affect their marital lives. Let me try to outline some of these; my comments are far from exhaustive. Depending upon the country of origin, the resident's adjustment to North America may be relatively straightforward or overwhelming. Examples of obstacles to be overcome include, for some, learning about and understanding a new culture or way of life; speaking and working in a new language; feeling isolated until acquaintances and friends are made; longing for and missing family members and familiar traditions; making dietary, housing, wearing apparel, and other life-style changes; studying and becoming comfortable with disease states and treatment methods that are specifically North American; preparing for and writing various licensure exams for IMGs; coming to terms with failure in first attempts at these exams; racial and ethnic discrimination by staff, fellow residents, and patients in the hospital setting; and striking a comfortable personal balance between letting go of some of the old ways and adopting some of the new.

Sometimes married IMGs are having more distress than they acknowledge, either to themselves or to program directors. Their work may begin to slip because of a host of personal and family problems, and their clinical supervisors may be concerned, especially if their performance and evaluations had been much better previously. They may not talk easily about what is going on at home, which is quite understandable given people's fears about disclosure in an unfamiliar culture and institution. These fears, coupled with more stringent and restrictive immigration regulations in North America at present, are very significant. Attitudes toward seeking and accepting professional help for marital problems will vary with one's country of origin. For those residents who do request help, therapists who are well trained and sensitive to issues of acculturation, medical marriages, and ethnocentric factors in the doctor–patient relationship must be available.

Finally, a significant number of IMGs intermarry during their residencies. I will not go into detail here because many of the statements about intermarriage and medical students made previously are applicable here. I only wish to emphasize that often these residents are coming to grips with monumental issues in their personal lives about which their clinical supervisors and program directors know nothing. I think that the more we can have communication and discussion between residents and teachers on subjects of personal stress, the better. Further, I predict that the more empathy and sensitivity that supervisors display toward their residents' personal lives, the more motivated, hardworking, and satisfied their trainees will be.

CONCLUSION

I want to conclude this chapter by emphasizing that there is a significant interplay between medical students' study or residents' work and their marriages. Because most couples are in the early years of their lives together, the process of rapid growth, change, and maturing corresponds with what is happening to them in medical school and residency as their professional identity is evolving. This can be both exciting and disconcerting, precipitating a fair amount of marital disequilibrium, as I have discussed in these pages. I turn in the next two chapters to the marriages of male and female physicians who have completed their training.

REFERENCES

1. Robert H. Coombs and Fawzy I. Fawzy, "The Effect of Marital Status on Stress in Medical School," *American Journal of Psychiatry* 139 (November 1982), 1490–1493.
2. John P. Tokarz, W. Bremer, and K. Peters, *Beyond Survival* (Chicago: American Medical Association, 1979).
3. Norman Cousins, "Internship: Preparation or Hazing?" *Journal of the American Medical Association* 245 (1981), 377.
4. David B. Reuben, "Psychologic Effects of Residency," *Southern Medical Journal* 76 (March 1983), 380–383.
5. Cynthia L. Janus, Samuel S. Janus, Susan Price, and David Adler, "Residents: The Pressure's on the Women," *Journal of the American Medical Women's Association* 38 (1983), 18–21.
6. Jack D. McCue, "The Distress of Internship," *New England Journal of Medicine* 312 (February 14, 1985), 449–452.
7. Paula S. Butterfield, "The Stress of Residency: A Review of the Literature," *Archives of Internal Medicine* 148 (June 1988), 1428–1435.
8. John M. Colford, Jr., and Stephen J. McPhee, "The Ravelled Sleeve of Care: Managing the Stresses of Residency Training," *Journal of the American Medical Association* 261 (February 10, 1989), 889–893.
9. Timothy B. McCall, "No Turning Back: A Blueprint for Residency Reform," *Journal of the American Medical Association* 261 (February 10, 1989), 909–910.
10. R. C. Friedman, Ronald Seymour Kornfeld, and T. J. Bigger, "Psychological Problems Associated with Sleep Deprivation in Interns," *Journal of Medical Education* 48 (1973), 436–441.
11. Michael J. Asken and David C. Raham, "Resident Performance and Sleep Deprivation: A Review," *Journal of Medical Education* 58 (May 1983), 382–388.
12. Paul Goldhammer and Michelle Farine, "Resident Night Call: Time for a Reappraisal," *Annals of the Royal College of Physicians and Surgeons of Canada* 18 (January 1985), 19–21.
13. Michael F. Myers, "When Hospital Doctors Labor to Exhaustion," *New York Times* (June 12, 1987), A22.
14. Leora R. Lewittes and Victor W. Marshall, "Fatigue and Concerns About Quality of Care Among Ontario Interns and Residents," *Canadian Medical Association Journal* 140 (January 1, 1989), 21–24.
15. Robert J. Valko and Paula J. Clayton, "Depression in the Internship," *Diseases of the Nervous System* 36 (1975), 26–29.
16. David C. Clark, Edgar Salazar-Grueso, Paula Grabler, and Jan Fawcett, "Predictors of

Depression During the First 6 Months of Internship," *American Journal of Psychiatry* 141 (1984), 1095–1098.

17. David B. Reuben, "Depressive Symptoms in Medical House Officers," *Archives of Internal Medicine* 145 (February 1985), 286–288.

18. Kirby Hsu and Victor Marshall, "Prevalence of Depression and Distress in a Large Sample of Canadian Residents, Interns, and Fellows," *American Journal of Psychiatry* 144 (December 1987), 1561–1566.

19. Elof G. Nelson and William F. Henry, "Psychosocial Factors Seen as Problems by Family Practice Residents and Their Spouses," *Journal of Family Practice* 6 (1978), 581–589.

20. Zebulon Taintor, Murray Morphy, Anne Seiden, and Eduardo Val, "Psychiatric Residency Training: Relationships and Value Development," *American Journal of Psychiatry* 140 (1983), 778–780.

21. Steven L. Schultz and Andrew T. Russell, "The Emotionally Disturbed Child Psychiatry Trainee," *Journal of the American Academy of Child Psychiatry* 23 (1984), 226–232.

22. Carol Landau, Stephanie Hall, Steven A. Wartman, and Michael B. Macko, "Stress in Social and Family Relationships During the Medical Residency," *Journal of Medical Education* 61 (August 1986), 654–660.

23. Merrijoy Kelner and Carolyn Rosenthal, "Postgraduate Medical Training, Stress, and Marriage," *Canadian Journal of Psychiatry* 31 (February 1986), 22–24.

24. David C. Spendlove, Barbara D. Reed, Neal Whitman, Martha L. Slattery, Thomas K. French, and Keith Horwood, "Marital Adjustment Among Housestaff and New Attorneys," *Academic Medicine* 65 (September 1990), 599–603.

25. Theresa Isomura and Michael F. Myers, "Women Doctors and Their Relationships," *British Columbia Medical Journal* 30 (May 1988), 332–335.

26. Glen O. Gabbard and Roy W. Menninger, "The Psychology of Postponement in the Medical Marriage," *Journal of the American Medical Association* 261 (April 28, 1989), 2378–2381.

27. Glen O. Gabbard, Roy W. Menninger, and Lolafaye Coyne, "Sources of Conflict in the Medical Marriage," *American Journal of Psychiatry* 144 (May 1987), 567–572.

28. Leanne D. Jolin, Paul Jolly, Jack Y. Krakower, and Robert Beran, "U.S. Medical School Finances," *Journal of the American Medical Association* 268 (September 2, 1992), 1149–1155.

29. Gloria J. Bazzoli and Steven D. Culler, "Factors Affecting Residents' Decisions to Moonlight," *Journal of Medical Education* 61 (October 1986), 797–802.

30. David O. Robinson, "The Medical Student Spouse Syndrome: Grief Reactions to the Clinical Years," *American Journal of Psychiatry* 135 (August 1978), 972–974.

31. Paul K. B. Dagg, "The Psychological Sequelae of Therapeutic Abortion—Denied and Completed," *American Journal of Psychiatry* 148 (May 1991), 578–585.

32. Nada L. Stotland, "The Myth of the Abortion Trauma Syndrome," *Journal of the American Medical Association* 268 (October 21, 1992), 2078–2079.

33. *Diagnostic and Statistical Manual of Mental Disorders*, third edition, revised (Washington, D.C.: American Psychiatric Association, 1987), 205–224.

34. Daniel B. Borenstein, "Should Physician Training Centers Offer Formal Psychiatric Assistance to House Officers? A Report on the Major Findings of a Prototype Program," *American Journal of Psychiatry* 142 (September 1985), 1053–1057.

35. Patrick H. Hughes, Scott E. Conrad, DeWitt C. Baldwin, Jr., Carla L. Storr, and David V. Sheehan, "Resident Substance Use in the United States," *Journal of the American Medical Association* 265 (1991), 2069–2073.

36. Patrick H. Hughes, DeWitt C. Baldwin, Jr., David V. Sheehan, Scott Conrad, and Carla

L. Storr, "Resident Physician Substance Use, by Specialty," *American Journal of Psychiatry* 149 (October 1992), 1348–1354.

37. Richard D. Aach, Donald E. Girard, Holly Humphrey, Jack D. McCue, David B. Reuben, Jay W. Smith, Lisa Wallenstein, and Jack Ginsburg, "Alcohol and Other Substance Abuse and Impairment Among Physicians in Residency Training," *Annals of Internal Medicine* 116 (February 1, 1992), 245–254.

38. R. Crawshaw, J. Bruce, P. Eraker, et al., "An Epidemic of Suicide Among Physicians on Probation," *Journal of the American Medical Association* 243 (1980), 1915–1917.

39. Howard B. Roback and Miles K. Crowder, "Psychiatric Resident Dismissal: A National Survey of Training Programs," *American Journal of Psychiatry* 146 (January 1989), 96–98.

40. Harry S. Jonas, Sylvia I. Etzel, and Barbara Barzansky, "Educational Programs in U.S. Medical Schools," *Journal of the American Medical Association* 268 (September 2, 1992), 1083–1090.

41. Henry K. Silver, "Medical Students and Medical School," *Journal of the American Medical Association* 247 (1982), 309–310.

42. Donna A. Rosenberg and Henry K. Silver, "Medical Student Abuse: An Unnecessary and Preventable Cause of Stress," *Journal of the American Medical Association* 251 (1984), 739–742.

43. "Effects of Medical Student Abuse Parallel Those of Child Abuse," *Psychiatric News* 26 (December 6, 1991), 4, 23.

44. Judith A. Richman, Joseph A. Flaherty, Kathleen M. Rospenda, and Michelle L. Christensen, "Mental Health Consequences and Correlates of Reported Medical Student Abuse," *Journal of the American Medical Association* 267 (1992), 692–694.

45. Egon Mayer, *Love and Tradition: Marriage Between Jews and Christians* (New York: Plenum Press, 1985), 119.

46. L. Belkin, "Many in Medicine See Rules Sapping Profession's Morale," *New York Times* (February 19, 1990), A1, A9.

47. N. Gibbs, "Sick and Tired," *Time* (July 31, 1989), 28–33.

48. Sherwyn Woods, personal communication, May 21, 1985.

49. Martin Goldberg, "Conjoint Therapy of Male Physicians and Their Wives," *Psychiatric Opinion* 12 (1975), 19–23.

50. Robert Krell and James E. Miles, "Marital Therapy of Couples in Which the Husband Is a Physician," *American Journal of Psychotherapy* 30 (1976), 267–275.

51. Michael Garvey and Vicente B. Tuason, "Physician Marriages," *Journal of Clinical Psychiatry* 40 (1979), 129–131.

52. James E. Miles, Robert Krell, and Tsung Y. Lin, "The Doctor's Wife: Mental Illness and Marital Patterns," *International Journal of Psychiatric Medicine* 6 (1975), 481–487.

53. Carla Fine, *Married to Medicine* (New York: Atheneum, 1981).

54. Esther M. Nitzberg, *Hippocrates' Handmaidens: Women Married to Physicians* (New York: Haworth, 1991).

55. Michael F. Myers, "The Female Physician and Her Marriage," *American Journal of Psychiatry* 141 (1984), 1386–1391.

56. Carol C. Nadelson and Malkah T. Notman, "The Woman Physician's Marriage," in *Medical Marriages,* ed. Glen O. Gabbard and Roy W. Menninger (Washington, D.C.: American Psychiatric Press, 1988), 79–88.

57. Gordon Parker and Roslyn Jones, "The Doctor's Husband," *British Journal of Medical Psychology* 54 (1981), 143–147.

58. Cynda Ann Johnson, Bruce E. Johnson, and Bruce S. Liese, "Dual-Doctor Marriages: The British Experience," *Journal of the American Medical Women's Association* 46 (September/October 1991), 155–159, 163.

59. Michael F. Myers, "The Abandoned Husband," *Medical Aspects of Human Sexuality* 18 (1984), 159–171.
60. Michael F. Myers, "Angry, Abandoned Husbands: Assessment and Treatment," *Marriage and Family Review* 9 (1985), 31–42.
61. W. Goode, "Theory of Role Strain," *American Sociological Review* 25 (1960), 283–299.
62. Frank A. Johnson and Colleen L. Johnson, "Role Strain in High-Commitment Career Women," *Journal of the American Academy of Psychoanalysis* 4 (1976), 13–36.
63. Michael F. Myers, "The Professional Woman as Patient: A Review and Appeal," *Canadian Journal of Psychiatry* 27 (1982), 236–240.
64. Michael F. Myers, "Marital Distress Among Resident Physicians," *Canadian Medical Association Journal* 134 (May 15, 1986), 1117–1118.
65. Nancy C. A. Roeske, "Stress and the Physician," *Psychiatric Annals* 11 (1981), 245–258.
66. Rosalind C. Barnett, Nancy L. Marshall, and Joseph H. Pleck, "Men's Multiple Roles and Their Relationship to Men's Psychological Distress," Working Paper No. 241, Wellesley College Center for Research on Women, 1991.
67. Maureen Sayres, Grace Wyshak, Geraldine Denterlein, Roberta Apfel, Eleanor Shore, and Daniel Federman, "Pregnancy During Residency," *New England Journal of Medicine* 314 (February 13, 1986), 418–423.
68. Paul D. Forman, "Parental Leave and Medical Careers," *Journal of the American Medical Association* 267 (February 5, 1992), 741.

Chapter Two

MALE PHYSICIAN MARRIAGES

How does a clinician begin to discuss the marriage problems of male doctors? Several authors have described their observations of physicians and their wives, both in the clinical setting and in surveys.[1-12] They have talked about the enormous pressures and stresses of medical work and their consequences on the personal and family lives of doctors. Most of the research has centered upon "traditional" medical marriages. This situation is rapidly changing in North America.

In a traditional medical marriage, the physician is the breadwinner and his wife is homemaker and mother to the children. His work is paid, hers unpaid. With our changing global economy and changing sex roles, there are fewer and fewer traditional medical marriages, except in families with young children (once the children are in school, many wives return to full- or part-time work outside the home). In a dual-career medical marriage, both the physician and his wife are working outside the home for pay, and usually homemaking and parenting are shared or delegated to others who are paid (nannies, housekeepers, day care, and so forth). In most dual-career marriages, the executive functions of running the home are done by the woman, and when the children are young, the woman's career involvement is less than that of her husband.

There is no "typical" male physician marriage any more than there is a "typical" marriage. Marital customs, roles, expectations, and disappointments are highly determined by one's ethnic and racial origin, one's religion, and the culture in which one was raised, as well as when one studied medicine, one's medical specialty, age at marriage, whom one married, and a host of other psychosocial factors. These are only a handful of the myriad variables that give all marriages a sense of uniqueness and mystery.

Having said this, however, there are common concerns and problem areas in the marriages of male doctors that cut across these variables and other demographic factors. What follows are several sections that describe problems; in these sections I discuss the surface complaints that one or both partners bring to therapy and my observations and clinical findings in assessing and treating maritally distressed doctors and their wives.

COMMUNICATION DIFFICULTIES

"We're not communicating." This concern is extremely common, if not universal, in troubled couples and can mean many different things, including not making the time to talk together as a twosome; not talking enough or at all to each other; talking only about superficial or "safe" topics; talking without getting the message across to each other; and talking that leads to tension, arguing, defensiveness, frustration, and withdrawal.

Doctors' wives, like women in general, are most apt to identify and become concerned about marital communication change or difficulty before their husbands. This seems to be a gender-specific difference between women and men. Historically, women have done the "worry work" of marriage, tending to the health of their marriages in much the same way that they have tended to their children, their homes, and their communities. More recently, with sex-role changes affecting marital dynamics, increasing numbers of male physicians, especially younger men, are beginning to talk about communication concerns in their marriages. These same men are more assertive and less embarrassed about reaching out for professional help.

Knowing how to communicate and how to communicate effectively in marriage is a goal that all of us hope to attain. But how do we achieve this goal? Is it an innate ability, an acquired and learned skill, or some mixture of "nature and nurture"? Are there fundamental differences between men and women in their abilities, their desires, and attempts to communicate, in general, and with each other? And more specifically, do doctors, given the nature of their personalities and the nature of their training and work, have particular types of communication problems in their marriages?

There are no easy answers to these questions, but my work as a psychiatrist treating troubled marriages, especially medical marriages, has been illuminating. People vary enormously in their ability to identify their needs and to communicate them clearly to their partners. Sager's description of the three different levels of communication in marriage—conscious and verbalized, conscious but not verbalized, and beyond awareness—is helpful.[13] Since the clearest and most direct form of communication, communication that is conscious and verbalized, is only one part (and a small part at that in some couples) of the exchange between partners, one can see how messages easily become distorted and misunderstood.

Let me explain these three levels of communication briefly. When we communicate at a conscious and verbalized level, we talk about matters that we are aware of and have no difficulty expressing to our spouses. This is easy, straightforward, and usually oriented toward goals and solving problems. Both partners should feel listened to and understood. There is a sense of comfort, achievement, and solidarity when the bulk of communication is like this.

The next level of communication, conscious but not verbalized, is more complicated. One or both of the marriage partners are aware of thoughts and feelings that they do not express. Why not? There may be several reasons. The individual may never have been very open or communicative (i.e., he or she is known to be a quiet, shy, or private person). Or he or she may have been raised in a home atmosphere that was not very expressive, or may have been criticized, scolded, or beaten for expressing feeling or opinion. Some people in marriage monitor or censor what they say because they have perceived or learned over the course of their relationship that some subjects precipitate strong emotion (crying, hurt, sadness, rage, guilt, anxiety, etc.) or frightening behavior (verbal retaliation, physical violence, sexual forcefulness, drinking, silent withdrawal, abandonment, etc.) in their spouse. Consequently, many issues never get talked about, and communication stays at a very superficial, polite, or prosaic level.

The third level, beyond awareness, is the most complicated. This is the "stuff" that we are not even aware of, and therefore we cannot discuss it. Because it is unconscious, we may get glimpses or fragments from our dreams—not always the actual content that we recall upon awakening, but certainly the themes or mood of our dreams (e.g., being perpetrator or victim of aggression, being lost, running away, feeling controlled or trapped, being sexually or emotionally involved with someone other than one's spouse). We may also get clues of unconscious and unexpressed feelings and ideas when we have had too much to drink (i.e., we lose our inhibitions and say things or behave in certain ways that do not occur otherwise). Sarcasm toward our spouses is often indicative of unconscious hostility that we are not aware of until we hear ourselves speak or are called on it.

Here is an example of a couple who came for marital therapy because of their concerns about communication:

Dr. M and Dr. B's chief complaint was that "we have major problems with communication—we can't discuss the weather without arguing." I asked each of them to explain and learned that Dr. M was a hematologist and Dr. B, his wife, was a psychologist. They met in graduate school when they were both working on their doctorates in psychology (Dr. M later decided to go to medical school and do a residency in hematology). Because of their training and experience in the behavioral sciences, they were especially frustrated and puzzled about their trouble communicating with each other.

In the early visits of marital therapy, I was struck by the degree of verbal competition that existed between Dr. M and Dr. B. They really did argue about almost everything. Although they complained of this, I was also aware that they enjoyed some of the verbal games they played with each other. Their respective vocabularies were dazzling, and it was a struggle for me not to get caught up in the intellectual volley of their talk. They were both very bright and skilled at holding their own on the minefield of marital communication.

My individual interviews with each of them had yielded important information that they were not sharing or had not shared with each other. For example, Dr. M's first girlfriend in high school became pregnant by him and had a therapeutic abortion, about which he felt guilty and ashamed. He had also had a psychotic experience, possibly drug induced, while in college in Israel and was hospitalized for a couple of weeks. Dr. B had herself had a therapeutic abortion in the past and had told no one except a close woman friend. She had cheated once on a very important exam and although she was never found out, she ruminated about this from time to time in a guilty and remorseful way. I wondered if much of their verbal sparring was a defense against a deeper level of communication and vulnerability. I floated this hunch before them in one particularly tense visit and asked each of them to consider disclosing some of the many feelings that they had discussed with me privately.

What followed was an exciting period of several weeks in which they talked more openly and deeply than they had ever done. They felt much closer, were certainly more affectionate with each other in my office, and noted that their sexual relationship had become more passionate and interesting. Their arguing was less frequent and less volatile.

After several conjoint visits, Dr. M announced that he had something quite frightening and embarrassing to bring up. He had had a dream about five days previously from which he awakened in a cold sweat. Just prior to awakening, he remembered touching the penis of one of his patients, a nine-year-old boy with leukemia. He was mortified and could not go back to sleep. He had not told his wife about the dream until recounting it in her presence in my office. She was very comforting and reassuring as he tearfully wondered aloud: "What's this mean? Am I gay? Am I a pedophile? Am I safe to practice medicine?" I asked him if anyone had ever touched him in a similar way when *he was a boy. He said no very quickly, then said, "Wait a minute!" and began to cry more. After a few minutes he recalled being fondled by a priest after assisting with Mass as an altar boy when he was "about eight or nine." Dr. B spontaneously said, "I think I know why you hate me to stimulate your penis with my hand during foreplay."*

This greatly condensed vignette describes how communication at a conscious and verbalized level was not clear and certainly not adequate for this highly functioning couple. Communication at a conscious but previously nonverbalized level led to a sense of relief, common purpose, problem solving, and enhanced intimacy. Communication at a previously unconscious level led to even more understanding and mutual sensitivity.

In order to understand more fully one's difficulty in marital communication, it helps to think about childhood and family dynamics. Many individuals who come for marital therapy have already begun to examine their parents' marriages. The reader may find the following internal dialogues familiar: "What are the similarities and differences between my marriage and my parents?" "In which ways do I identify with my father (or my mother) in expressing feelings?" "Did they fight a lot?" "Do we fight a lot?" (If yes, "I learned it from them, they were my role models." Or if no, "I hated their fighting, I vowed to not fight in my marriage at all costs.") "Were they openly affectionate toward each other?" ("No, but I wish they were. I want that in my marriage. I try to be affectionate but it's not easy for me." "My father turned to alcohol when he was under stress. I see myself doing the same thing— I have to watch it.")

These introspective questions have insight and change as their goal. They arise from a given psychodynamic that all human beings are shaped, for better or for worse, by a biopsychosocial matrix of factors that they then bring into their marriages. These questions are directed at the self, and this is important, because until a person is able to do this honestly and courageously, he or she cannot communicate maturely and constructively in marriage.

What are the ways in which men and women in marriages communicate their needs differently? As a general rule, men are not in touch with their feelings as completely or as accurately as women. Their feelings are also more likely to be hidden, not only from themselves, but from their wives and others. Many wives describe loneliness in marriage. They complain either that their husbands do not talk to them enough (a quantitative issue), or that their husbands do not share private thoughts and feelings (a qualitative issue). Indeed many women feel they are forever second-guessing or "reading between the lines" with their husbands.

This is not to say that men who are not "talkers" do not communicate in marriage. If one looks at some of the behavioral patterns of men in marriages—overwork, emotional withholding, sexual harassment and demandingness, and physical violence—one sees that there is a lot being communicated. One also comes to appreciate the tremendous power and control that are contained in these behaviors. But because it is largely unconscious, or when conscious is certainly oblique, most couples cannot begin to decipher it. Regretfully, most men (and their wives) in these marriages cannot look back at their fathers' communicating styles as being any clearer or more exemplary.

Dr. Deborah Tannen, author of *You Just Don't Understand: Women and Men in Conversation* and professor of linguistics at Georgetown University, has studied differing conversational styles in men and women.[14] She postulates that many frictions arise because boys and girls grow up in what are essentially different cultures, so that talk between women and men is cross-cultural communication. Her observations of asymmetries in speech, interruptions in conversation, gossip, and silence are splendid and go a long way toward reassuring men and women in marriage that they are not crazy or wrong, just different.

Finally, what about male doctors? In addition to the generic issues regarding marital communication difficulties and gender-specific differences already discussed, is there anything that can be concluded about how we communicate in our marriages? Many of us do not set aside the time for talk and relaxation in our marriages. We feel that our work—our patients, our hospital committee meetings, our students, our research, our journal reading, our career advancement—is more important, that our wives must understand, and that our marriages will flourish by spirit alone. Many doctors expect their wives to be "strong," which means they must be capable of everything from raising the children largely unassisted to repairing the roof! And most emphatically, we expect them to never complain. Let me illustrate this with a common example from my practice.

Mrs. R was referred to me by her family doctor, Dr. W, because of anxiety and depressive symptoms. Dr. W told me over the phone that he thought her symptoms were largely a result of her marriage. Her husband was a busy and highly respected neurologist "whose whole life is medicine." Dr. W felt that Mrs. R was overstressed—she was not only busy running the home and looking after four children but also busy tending to Dr. R's aged and infirm mother, who lived next door. When I asked Dr. W if Dr. R might come with his wife, he intimated that Dr. R would never acknowledge a marital problem, let alone marital therapy.

Mrs. R came to see me alone and, indeed, she was having a lot of difficulty coping with everything. She was not clinically depressed but was afraid of becoming so because her mother had a recurrent depressive illness that had required hospitalization and shock treatments. She was also very lonely and very unassertive in her marriage—she didn't martyr herself in a self-pitying or attention-seeking way, but she did put herself down constantly. She hadn't told her husband she had come to see me. She said, "I don't want to bother him, and I don't want him to think less of me."

I worked alone with Mrs. R for a while, and she began to feel a lot better about herself. She then decided to tell her husband she was seeing me. He didn't react as negatively as she had expected. When I expressed my desire to meet with him, she asked him, and again to her surprise he agreed to come in. My visit with him went well, and he felt fine about returning for a few visits with his wife to talk about their relationship. He had done a lot of thinking about his life and his work and was ready to make some changes, changes that were long overdue in both their opinions.

Most male doctors, but not all, have compulsive personalities—or at least compulsive traits.[15] Being perfectionistic, orderly, moral, and conscientious is adaptive and necessary for the practice of medicine. But being rigid, emotionally inhibited, overdutiful, and unable to relax easily does not make one a tremendously exciting husband. Indeed, Ellis and Inbody have described seven attributes in physicians that serve them well professionally but can become liabilities in family life: control, perfectionism, withholding of anger, competitiveness, dedication, perennial caretaker, and emotional remoteness.[16]

Physicians with severely compulsive personalities do not communicate easily with their wives and tend to be emotionally isolated. They talk in terms of "thoughts," not "feelings"; they are pedantic and tend to lecture their wives; their talk has a superior, self-righteous, and arrogant quality that, despite its often being a defense against underlying anxiety and insecurity, is terribly off-putting and alienating in marriage. Their wives classically are completely opposite—outgoing, dynamic, emotionally ranging—and their marriages have been typed elsewhere as "love-sick" wife–"cold-sick" husband.[17]

This is the extreme and the stereotype. In reality, most male physicians whose marriages are in trouble are deeply concerned about the degree of unhappiness experienced by their wives, their children, and themselves. Most of these physicians are very conscious of overworking and feel guilty—they have difficulty saying no—and often feel they are on a treadmill. Most admit to having trouble relaxing. Most are very interested in learning new and more efficient ways of communicating and take an active and concerted interest in marital therapy. And many bemoan the lack of teaching about marriage in medical school and/or the de-emphasis on marital health and function during residency training.

OVERWORK

This is a common problem area in marriages of male doctors. It is almost always a complaint initially recognized and aired by wives about their physician husbands. It is the rare male physician who does not react defensively when first charged with working too hard. The defensiveness is fully comprehensible—medicine is not a nine-to-five job; people get sick and cannot gear their injuries and fevers to a regular schedule; one does have to see more patients if office overheads continue to rise; one does have to attend a certain number of staff meetings and serve on committees; the mortgage does have to be paid; and children's college fees are not getting any lower. Unfortunately, many couples do not get beyond this point when trying to discuss overwork. What these wives don't get a chance to talk about are their feelings of loneliness; their nostalgic longing for the "young and carefree man I married"; their sense of marital intimacy slowly slipping away; and in some women, their growing and frightening attraction to alcohol, drugs, or other men.

It has been documented that the ratings on marital satisfaction indices are at their lowest during the childbearing and early child-rearing years when children are not yet in school. For male doctors, these years often correspond with residency and early practice years. It is at this time that young male physicians are mainly outer directed—completing training, establishing a practice, repaying education debts, developing a positive and solid image in the medical community, and affirming their inner sense of professional confidence. In traditional marriages, wives are home during these years; their responsibilities center around raising the children, running the household, and serving the community. Their work is unpaid and too often unappreciated. These women have high rates of depression.

Increasing numbers of wives of male doctors are working outside the home, some out of economic necessity as well as personal needs and others because of their own careers. Despite differences in income between men and women, this shift is enabling many male physicians to work fewer hours per week, to bear less than full responsibility for earning the money, and most importantly to take a more active role in raising their children. This change begins to address the male physician overwork syndrome, but with both partners working outside the home, couples must guard against not having enough time together and short-changing each other.

Newly retired male physicians may present with a marital problem also based in overwork, but overwork in a historical sense. These couples over the years have made a compromise: He has devoted his life to medicine, and she has devoted her life to the children, the home, friends, individual interests, and now the grandchildren. He has a lot of free time on his hands and wants to spend more time with his wife while adapting to retirement and trying out new interests. When she is busy with her friends and activities, he feels hurt and rejected.

Is overwork always a cause of marital discord, or can it be the result? For some, work has become an escape from marital unhappiness. And most doctors in this situation secretly know it. They have not loved their wives for some time but are coping as best as they can. They are aware that they feel stimulated at work, take assurance in being liked and respected by their patients, and feel confident and good about themselves as doctors. As husbands, and often as fathers, they feel they have failed. They are ashamed and embarrassed to reach out for professional help—and usually tell themselves it wouldn't help anyway. Divorce is no solution; it is seen as a cop-out and a relinquishing of one's responsibilities as a man. Some consider having an affair but rule that out ("Do I really need more hassle and more guilt?"). Only work, and more work, is ennobling.

Dr. S admitted that he would never have come to see me as a patient had I not met him in a different capacity a year earlier. His son, Kevin, a second-year medical student, had come to see me at that time because he was contemplating dropping out of medical school and the dean had suggested he consult a psychiatrist before doing so. Kevin was actually quite depressed, and in order to obtain collaborative information I interviewed Dr. and Mrs. S.

When Dr. S returned on his own a year later his words were, "I'm not sure why I'm here or even if you can help me, but one thing I'm sure about is that I don't want anyone giving me any advice about what to do." Dr. S went on to tell me about his life, especially his married life, for the remainder of the visit. His story got sadder by the minute. He described years of increasing emotional distance between himself and his wife, coupled with a work pace that would have exhausted a twenty-year-old. Their marriage was a charade in many respects. He and his wife felt it necessary to keep up a facade of happiness for their children and for the sake of his position as a department head at the medical school. Their sexual relationship had ended fifteen years earlier.

Dr. S was very bottled up. I'm sure he could have talked for hours. At the end of the hour, I suggested we meet again, a visit at a time, depending on his wishes. This we did. I didn't give him any advice! Together we created the context in which he could talk freely and openly, something he had not been able to do with his male friends.

I want to conclude this section by making a distinction between simple overwork in physicians and workaholism. My comments thus far have been mainly about the former, that is, male physicians who overwork and have marital problems. They are much more common than physicians suffering from workaholism. Killinger defines a workaholic as a person who is addicted to power and control, not necessarily to the love of his or her work per se.[18] It represents a compulsive drive to gain approval and success because of underlying anxieties and insecurities. Workaholism is most manifest when work or work-related projects take over a person's life—nothing else matters. Unlike physicians who simply overwork, these individuals lack a balance of work, play, and family time in their lives. There is a high risk of addiction to alcohol or other drugs, impaired judgment, burnout, depression, marital breakdown, and suicide. Needless to say, these physicians are a worrisome group who can fall through the cracks and not receive psychiatric or psychological help.

ALCOHOL ABUSE

Excessive use of alcohol by the physician and/or his wife is frequently associated with marital conflict and unhappiness. In most couples, alcohol abuse is the primary problem that causes marital strain. The marital strain, in turn, may aggravate the drinking problem, but rarely does primary marital discord produce alcohol abuse *de novo*. The main situation in which marital problems *antedate* excessive drinking is when one or both partners drink excessively and usually symptomatically during acute marital crises. This is almost always only a short-term situation, such as a marital crisis precipitated by very recent disclosure of an extramarital affair.

Vulnerability to alcoholism is well documented in physicians,[9,19–22] and most medical communities now have physician well-being committees and treatment centers for impaired doctors. [23–25] Unfortunately, by the time many physicians accept their drinking problem and begin treatment, their marriages and family life are a shambles. Indeed, threatened or actual separation may be one of the major motivators in physicians coming to terms with the gravity of their alcohol problem.

In marriages where neither partner is alcohol dependent, regular and frequent use of alcohol can still adversely affect marital communication, solidarity, and intimacy. Wives of such physicians complain of how a couple of drinks in the evening affect their husbands' behavior: "He gets sleepy and withdrawn; it's impossible to have a conversation." "It's the sarcasm and belligerence that I hate—the only time he expresses anything negative about me is when he's been drinking." "Alcohol on his breath is the biggest turn-off, and ironically, that's the only time he approaches me sexually anymore." "He's only hit me when he's been drinking."

Making a diagnosis of alcohol dependence can be very difficult because of denial and minimizing by the physician himself and sometimes in collusion with his wife. One also attempts, in conducting a thorough psychiatric assessment of individuals requesting marital therapy, to rule out (and treat, if present) underlying illnesses such as anxiety states, phobic disorders, mood disorders, and the like. In general, individuals cannot work together in marital therapy if one or both are psychiatrically ill or continue to do a lot of drinking. The following is an example of a couple in which a host of defenses and emotions (denial, rationalizing, collusion, shame, and fear of exposure) were operating in both the impaired physician and his wife.[26]

Dr. and Mrs. A came to see me at the urging of their twenty-three-year-old son, who was called to the family home after Dr. A had physically assaulted his wife. Dr. A had driven home at four a.m. intoxicated after a late poker game with several other doctors. He awakened his wife after smashing into the garage door, which he thought was open. Dr. A struck his wife with his fist (resulting in a black eye) when she confronted him about drinking and driving. Although Dr. A had at least a ten-year history of an established drinking problem with morning shakes, alcoholic blackouts, and one warning for impaired driving, he had never sought help. Likewise, Mrs. A had never spoken to her family physician or gone to Alanon despite repeated exhortations from her four adult children.

SELF-MEDICATION

The phenomenon of drug-taking in doctors is well known and well researched.[20–25,27–31] The range of drugs abused is wide (narcotic analgesics, barbiturates, benzodiazepines, amphetamines, and occasionally appetite suppressants and CNS stimulants like Ritalin) and is classically due to at least three factors: personal vulnerability,[32] excessive work stress (which produces anxiety, self-doubt, fatigue, sleeplessness, etc.), and easy availability of drugs on the job. The most common street drugs that doctors use are marijuana, hashish, and cocaine. The relevance of drug abuse to marriage is critical because its consequences range from communication difficulties when the doctor is impaired to marital estrangement and social ostracism if the doctor loses his license to practice. As in the case of alcoholism in doctors, the problem of drug abuse may become circular when well advanced, but, in general, it is the drug-taking that leads to marital stress rather than the other way around.

Many physicians will volunteer their use of drugs because they are concerned, not just about their self-administration of drugs, but about their need for medication of any sort. They may feel ashamed and guilty; they may fear reprisals. They may not have told their wives, who in turn know absolutely nothing. But many wives suspect that something has been amiss for some time. Impaired physicians underestimate how much their drug-taking secret is antithetical to the self-disclosure that is a crucial ingredient in fostering marital intimacy. As with alcohol abuse, marital therapy cannot proceed until the drug problem is treated.

> Dr. and Mrs. M came requesting marital therapy. They both admitted in the first few minutes of the visit that their situation was complicated. Dr. M said, "I'm an alcoholic. I have been for ten years. I can't deny it any longer. Alcohol is killing me, and my family." Mrs. M said, "And I take too many pills. I'm hooked on Valium and I have been for at least a year. I want to get off them." Both went on to describe a marriage that they both agreed was a close second to the marriage of George and Martha in Who's Afraid of Virginia Woolf?
>
> With the assistance of our local impaired-physician committee, I arranged to have Dr. M admitted for residential treatment of his alcoholism. At the same time, Mrs. M was admitted to a drug rehabilitation center for women. They both completed the first phase of treatment as inpatients and were then enrolled in their respective programs as outpatients. The three of us then began marital work, which largely focused on problems that had been there for years but were never addressed or resolved because of the interference of alcohol and drugs.

UNDIAGNOSED DEPRESSION

Depression can be both a cause and a result of marital difficulty. Doctors are as vulnerable to depression as anyone, and yet many physicians do not get adequate care and treatment. They may not recognize the symptoms in themselves, or when they do, they play them down. If and when they reach out for help, those who treat them may miss the diagnosis or underdiagnose. Depression in doctors lurks behind many cases of overwork, general fatigue, somatization disorders, burnout, alcoholism, and drug abuse.

Dr. F, who was a family physician and a former student of mine, called me to ask my opinion about a patient of his who was also a family physician in a nearby community. Dr. F queried whether his patient might be depressed, even though the man didn't feel depressed and bristled at the suggestion of depression. Dr. F's concern centered around his patient's increasing physical symptoms over the previous six months, symptoms that affected almost every system of his body and brought him into the office at least once every two weeks. He had had every blood test imaginable, X rays, and scans and had been assessed by a general internist, a cardiologist, a neurologist, and a urologist. Nothing organic could be found, and the patient really felt no better.

There were two other reasons why Dr. F suspected depression in his patient. The man's wife was also a patient of Dr. F's, and she had frequently complained over the years about her marriage, how hard her husband worked, and how he rarely took a proper vacation. Second, she had been in recently with genital herpes. She told Dr. F that she had been having an affair the previous year and knew she had contracted it from the man she was seeing. She was certain her husband didn't know. Dr. F was not so certain and wondered if this unspoken change in their marriage could be contributing to his patient's symptoms.

I agreed totally with his hunches. I urged him to take a firmer but kind approach to the man, explaining to him that he felt strongly that this might be a type of depression, and to arrange a consultation with a psychiatrist. This is what he did—his patient agreed, albeit tentatively, to see a psychiatrist, who diagnosed depression, started him on an antidepressant, and later referred the man and his wife to a psychologist for marital therapy.

Some depressed doctors who are able to recognize their mood change are too embarrassed to consult a psychiatrist. They feel they have failed, that they are "lesser men," that they are weak, that they can no longer compete. Too many physicians, like the lay public, continue to believe that depression represents a weakness of will, a moral failing, or a mark of imperfection.[33] Some have little to no respect for psychiatrists and cannot envision a psychiatrist being of any help. They may feel that the psychiatrist will judge them, will not understand, or will gloat over their distress. Many have outdated or narrow ideas about what psychiatrists actually do. They do not have an understanding of the sophistication and efficacy of modern psychiatry.

Over the years, I have seen and treated many depressed male physicians whose ticket of admission was a problem marriage. These men would not have come initially for individual treatment. There are many possible reasons for this: Admitting to needing psychiatric help is not easy for most people, including doctors; coming for marital therapy is more socially acceptable; coming together is a way to save face; seeing a marital "counselor" is less threatening than seeing a "psychiatrist"; and coming together enables the physician-patient to focus more on "the relationship" or his wife and less on himself until he is ready to do so.

There are important implications for the physician-husband when it is his wife who is depressed. One must always keep in mind that depressions have biological, psychological, and social determinants. The contributing weight of these three factors varies markedly from one person to the next. Historically, doctors' wives, like women in general but perhaps even more so, have been treated in isolation from their husbands. The treatment has been either very biologically focused, with sole reliance on medications, or very psychoanalytically based, with the woman remaining in long-term individual therapy.

When the wife of a doctor is clinically depressed, I feel that it is extremely important, if not essential, that her husband be interviewed. And he must be approached and assessed with support and objectivity as one would interview the husband of any depressed female patient. Too often psychiatrists, particularly male psychiatrists in smaller or tightly knit medical communities, do not involve the husbands. This might happen because they may feel uncomfortable with physicians and physicians' spouses as patients; they may know the physician-husband personally and feel that chatting in the hospital corridor or at the gym is adequate; their diagnostic and therapeutic approach to depressed patients does not include marital dynamics; or they themselves lack insight into their own marriages and deny depression in their wives or perhaps themselves.

Here is an example that illustrates my point quite boldly.

When Dr. O, a senior psychiatrist in our city, called to ask me if I would see his wife, these were his words: "She's really quite depressed—she has early morning wakening, anorexia, a weight loss of ten pounds, and no libido— I don't think she's suicidal, but there is manic-depressive illness in her family." I felt as though I was talking to this poor woman's family doctor, not her husband! I told him that I would be quite happy to see her, and I also told him I would want to meet with him at some point after my first visit with her. He quickly agreed and suggested lunch. I said no, that I'd set up a visit at my office.

My visit with Mrs. O went very well. She was indeed quite depressed and needed to go back on an antidepressant. She had a recurrent depressive illness and had seen two other psychiatrists in the past. She saw one of them on and off for five years—this man had never met or talked to Dr. O. The second psychiatrist worked with her for two years. When I asked her if he had met Dr. O, she said: "Yes, my husband and I saw him together once. He explained why he thought I got depressed, then my husband explained why he thought I got depressed, then the two of them discussed me and debated what antidepressant to put me on."

My interview with Dr. O also went very well, which I had not anticipated. After our talk on the phone and my knowledge of his one previous visit with his wife's former psychiatrist, I hadn't expected that I would be able to "reach" him. Although he was very clinical in the first few minutes of our session together, he dropped this very quickly as I talked with him the way I talk to any husband whose wife is and has been depressed a lot. This was very therapeutic for him, because he had a lot to talk about. He resented his wife's illness because they missed out on a lot of things when she was depressed. He had a lot of sadness about this also, because their life together before she became ill was so full of joy and companionship. He also worried about her a lot. Her brother and one of her grandfathers had committed suicide. I saw him again, for several visits actually, which helped not only him but also his wife.

Many physicians contribute to their wives' depressions by working too hard; by not striking a healthy balance between their work and personal lives; by not being emotionally available or supportive at home; by not assisting with looking after the children and doing their share of the chores; by not being complimentary and affectionate; or by not being their wife's life companion and "best friend." Discussing these issues is one of the ways the eclectic psychiatrist approaches depression in doctors' wives. Another way is psychoeducative (i.e., offering up-to-date information about depression and its management to physicians whose wives are very seriously depressed and on antidepressants). This approach also includes supportive psychotherapy for the doctor (and the children), because living with someone who is very depressed may be confusing, frightening, exhausting, and demoralizing until improvement begins.

Something that has been increasingly common in physicians over the past ten years is unhappiness and disillusionment with medical practice. This can contribute to clinical depression in doctors, or it may be confused with it. There may be associated symptoms of morbid self-absorption, feelings of bitterness, hostility, irritability, negative thinking, withdrawal, and extreme sensitivity—all of which may be very difficult for the doctor's wife and children. This demoralization seems to have many factors: increasing loss of autonomy in today's physicians, residual financial indebtedness from long years of education, complicated reimbursement procedures for one's work, conflict with insurance companies, inevitable movement toward managed care, lawsuits, and ever-escalating malpractice insurance rates.

One final point I want to make about depression in physicians and/or their wives is the tendency in some medical marriages for the physician to diagnose and treat. In other words, the physician concludes that he is depressed and starts taking an antidepressant, or he puts his wife on antidepressants. How commonly physicians treat depression in their wives is not known, but a recent and more general questionnaire survey of physicians showed that 83% of respondents had prescribed medication for a family member.[34] Since the advent of newer and "cleaner" antidepressants over the past few years, I am seeing increasing numbers of physicians who are treating themselves and family members with anti-depressants—sometimes with adverse consequences, as shown below.

One weekend when I was on call, I received a consultation request from the emergency room physician about a woman who had been brought in by the police. She had been apprehended for protesting in the nude in front of a supermarket about "toxic chemicals" being used by management to deceive the public about the freshness of their fruits and vegetables. She had bitten one of the police officers, was shouting profanities, and was talking constantly. I assessed her as being in a manic state and gave her some sedation while I continued to learn what had happened. She had no previous history of psychiatric illness, but her mother suffered from bipolar (manic-depressive) illness. She wouldn't talk to me, but I managed to reach her husband, an internist, who was out of the country at a medical meeting. When I explained to him about his wife's condition, he became very panicky and started to cry. He told me that she had been drinking a lot since her hysterectomy a year earlier and was quite depressed. He had given her some antidepressant samples three weeks earlier, and she began to feel better in about ten days. He felt terribly guilty about treating her and not insisting that she go to her own physician.

SEXUAL PROBLEMS

There are many different types of sexual concerns that physicians and their wives express in treatment: disorders of sexual desire, disorders of sexual arousal (erectile difficulty in men and lubrication difficulties in women), disorders of orgasm (premature and retarded ejaculation in men and orgasmic inhibition in women), extramarital sexual activity, and sexual orientation conflicts. To my knowledge, there is no greater incidence of sexual problems in doctors' marriages than there is in the general population.

Let me focus on a few of these concerns. Disorders of sexual desire in one or both partners are particularly important in doctors' marriages. Many male physicians, despite their protestations to the contrary, sublimate a great deal of their sexual energy into their work (and sometimes into vigorous sports). Their wives complain of a decrease in frequency of love making or of sexual activity that is devoid of feeling and intimacy. The latter may range from being hurried, brief, and somewhat mechanical to meticulous and methodical—both extremes less than ideal.

Often there is very little sexual communication, which should not be too surprising. Most couples do not easily discuss their sexual relationship. I do not believe that doctors are any more comfortable discussing sex with their spouses or partners than are laypersons. Despite physicians' medical understanding of sexuality, this knowledge generally is very biomedically skewed. Any comfort and facility that they have with their own sexuality is almost totally a reflection of their personal life experience, not what they've learned in lectures, textbooks, and clinical practice. The raunchy intern or resident "bedding all the nurses on Five East" is largely a Hollywood stereotype—many doctors have not had huge amounts of sexual experience with many different partners before marriage. And those who have are not necessarily more competent or more sensitive lovers. Learning to love maturely is more complicated than that.

Sometimes harbored within the hardworking and dedicated physician who is exhausted in the evening and "too tired" to make love is a disorder of sexual desire. Exhaustion from demanding patients and long working days may camouflage it. Behind the problem of sexual desire may be a lack of sexual confidence and sexual self-esteem that goes back many, many years to adolescence or early adulthood. Superimposed on this may be unexpressed marital slights, hurts, and resentments. All of these conditions may be unrecognized and unconscious. Without therapy, this situation may continue indefinitely.

Dr. E and his wife, Dr. L, came for marital therapy because of a sexual concern that they both felt, but it was Dr. L who pushed for professional help. She started the interview: "We're here because we hardly make love anymore.

For some reason or other, Jerry's shut down sexually. He never approaches me anymore, and I've stopped approaching him—I can only take so much rejection. We're beginning to discuss having children, and there's no way I want to start a family unless we get back on track sexually." Dr. E responded with, "I'm not happy to be here; this is Janice's idea, not mine. I consider sex a very private matter, and—no offense to you, Doctor Myers—I think we can take care of this ourselves." I attempted to reassure Dr. E as best I could and then proceeded to assess their situation with them in a very low-key and nonthreatening manner. There certainly had been a change in their sexual relationship, which was fine in the beginning. They made love a lot, and both enjoyed it then. Only when Dr. E left residency and was establishing his private practice did their lovemaking fall off. Neither of them could think of other problems that were affecting their marriage.

In my individual visit with Dr. E I learned that sex had never played a very important part in his life. He masturbated occasionally and had been sexual with other women a few times before he met his wife, but he had not had a sustained relationship, sexual or otherwise, with anyone. He had found himself quite preoccupied with his work and his garden. He said he often just didn't feel like making love. He had no complaints whatsoever about his wife: "I find her as sexy and as attractive as the day we met." He also didn't feel that he was withdrawing from her because he was angry.

In my visit with Dr. L I learned that, compared to her husband, she had had much more sexual experience, both in terms of the number of partners and in terms of how long she had been involved with someone. She also really enjoyed sex and saw it as an essential form of communication in a marriage. She also admitted that her self-esteem and sense of attractiveness had really slipped because the frequency of sex with her husband had decreased. She also admitted that she was angry at him "for being so lazy."

The three of us worked together, and their sexual relationship improved quickly. Unlike many couples with this type of concern, there were not a lot of conflicts causing the problem of sexual desire—or as a result of the problem of sexual desire. Dr. E simply needed to prioritize his life a bit differently, think more about marital sex, and make overtures to his wife more regularly. It also helped him to know how insecure his wife began to feel when they went long periods without making love. He hadn't known that. I also urged Dr. L to return to making sexual advances in order to give balance to their sexual life together.

In many marriages, each partner blames the other for a lack of sexual desire or for not initiating sex often enough. This can be very confusing. In Western society, it is easier—that is, more socially acceptable—for women to admit to a change in or loss of interest in sex. Many men, including male physicians, have difficulty admitting their lack of interest in sex to themselves and to others. Men are expected to be hot-blooded and libidinous creatures well into their nineties. I have seen a number of physicians in therapy over the years whose minimal interest in sex was very well concealed. They saw their wives as sexually dysfunctional and blamed them—any effort or overture on their wives' initiative was derided or belittled. They saw themselves as always sexually ready, which they were, but in a childlike, demanding, or petulant way that only reinforced their wives' retreat and withdrawal. As time went on their sexual relationship deteriorated to a tug-of-war, full of anxiety, tension, and anger. Sex became a chore and an act of compliance—no longer were they "making love."

Let me turn now to the subject of extramarital sexual activity. I will confine my comments to those situations in which the behavior is "ego dystonic," that is, behavior that causes upset (anxiety, depression, guilt) in the individual. Some physicians seek help when they have become involved with someone else and their wives do not know about their involvement. Another situation exists when a man has disclosed the outside relationship to his wife (or she has found out and confronted him), and this knowledge precipitates an acute and rapidly escalating marital crisis. Most of these men are quite surprised, if not alarmed, at their situation. Rarely are they fully in touch with the degree of vulnerability, personal loneliness, and marital distance that has preceded their meeting and falling in love with the other person.

Dr. P called to make an appointment with me "ASAP." In that first visit he told me that two months earlier, while attending his twentieth-year high school reunion, he had spent most of the weekend in bed with his "high school sweetheart." Dr. P was married and the father of three children. Because his wife had come from another part of the country, she did not accompany him on his journey to the reunion weekend. Upon seeing his former girlfriend, Pam, who was divorced from her husband, Dr. P was overcome with old feelings "that had never really gone away." "She looked even more beautiful than she was in high school," he stated.

Dr. P had done a lot of reflecting before coming to see me. He had spoken to Pam several times over the phone since he returned home from the weekend. Although she was very interested and willing to see him again, she was also adamant that she was not going to become a "homewrecker." She was glad that he was going for therapy. Dr. P, trying not to compare the excitement and thrill of a "dirty weekend" with his marriage of fifteen years, complained that he and his wife were not as close as he would like. It was refreshing to hear that he did not entirely blame his wife for being so busy with the kids, the home, and her community work—he also implicated himself for working nonstop for many years and not taking "getaway" weekends with his wife. Their lovemaking had suffered, not in frequency, but in its depth and fulfillment. He also found himself feeling rather lonely in his marriage. More and more he was sitting on things, even mundane matters, and this made him feel quite isolated. I also felt that his life was far too serious (he laughingly agreed) and that he needed more time for leisure and fun, both with his wife and on his own.

I only had three visits with Dr. P. He was able to open up more to his wife and talk about the boredom and loneliness he was feeling in the marriage. She seemed to be able to accept this and to join him in making efforts to improve things. They did not need marital therapy.

Here is an example of another couple struggling with an extramarital relationship, in this case precipitated by competing commitments in the marriage:

Dr. Brown and Mrs. Brown came to see me because they were in crisis— he had recently ended a six-month affair with a woman from his triathalon group. He wanted to remain in his marriage, and he wanted marital therapy to try to get things back on track. Mrs. Brown was not so sure if she wanted to stay married or to work on things with her husband; she was very hurt, very angry, and very mistrustful of her husband's motives.

Dr. Brown complained that there was no companionship or intimacy in his marriage and speculated that this was how and why he got involved with someone else. He was resentful that his wife was working so many weekend shifts (she was a nurse), that she was busy with night school two evenings a week, that she had so much studying to do, that their two children and their activities seemed to take priority over him or their relationship, and that she only felt like sex about once a month. Mrs. Brown argued that her husband was as busy or busier than she—that he worked roughly twelve-hour days at the hospital and his office, that he was detached and numb at home, that he was on too many work-related committees and was out many of the evenings that she was home, and that he was obsessed with running, cycling, and swimming, all of which she found "narcissistic and boringly healthy." Although she was not a smoker, she occasionally bought a pack and loved to light up a cigarette after dinner and blow smoke his way. Fortunately, all three of us found this funny when she brought it up in the first visit. I made a mental note of this, because I thought it meant a good prognosis for the two of them—and I was right; they did very well with marital therapy.

Before making any immediate decision about his marriage, the physician should consult a psychiatrist. Therapeutic work with a well-trained and experienced professional will serve several purposes: It will alleviate some of the anxiety and distress in both parties; shed light on whether the physician is depressed and, if so, advise and assist with treatment; begin to uncover some of the underlying determinants of the marital malaise; clarify whether the marriage is viable; facilitate decision making that is sound and appropriate; and most importantly, if the decision is to separate, provide sustenance and care to all family members (or assist with referrals to other professionals).

Another aspect of extramarital sexual activity in male physicians that I wish to touch on briefly is sexual involvement with patients. (I will discuss this subject in more detail in Chapter Seven.) This is an important subject that is only recently being talked about and studied vigorously.[35-39] In keeping with the theme of this chapter, the married male physician, let me focus on only one facet of this problem, that is, the symptomatic doctor who has fallen in love with and/or become sexual with one of his female patients. I will not discuss the character-disordered doctor who has become sexual with a patient (or patients, since recidivism in this type is common), because these men are very different—they deny or lie about their behavior, are not symptomatic, and are best managed by ethics committees, licensing bodies, and the courts.

The symptomatic married physician who has become involved with a patient is in double jeopardy; not only is his marital equilibrium upset by the outside relationship, but his choice of person is inappropriate and unethical. He has to contend with added feelings of shame and disapproval on top of already dysphoric emotions associated with a marital crisis. Consequently, some of these men are already, or become, quite ill. Unfortunately, many do not reach out for professional help because of fear and self-loathing. They also assume that the treating psychiatrist will be horrified and disgusted. These assumptions only enhance their panic and isolation. Some commit suicide. Needless to say, this is an area that needs immediate attention during undergraduate and postgraduate medical education because it so pointedly crystallizes the vulnerability of physicians throughout their professional lives. Likewise, psychiatric residents need teaching on this subject and experience in treating physicians who are psychiatrically distressed.

Finally, what about sexual orientation conflict in married male doctors? Homosexual conflict certainly exists in some physicians and may be a concern that a doctor brings to therapy. Examples of concerns may include any of the following: intermittent yet troubling homosexual dreams with no homosexual feelings, thoughts, or desires during waking hours; homosexual thoughts and desires when one's wife is pregnant; occasional use of homosexual imagery during masturbation; memories of having been sexually abused as a child; feelings of sexual arousal when physically examining certain male patients; an inner acceptance of being gay coupled with a waning sexual desire for one's wife; and a recent extramarital relationship with another man.

Homosexual feelings, thoughts, and desires are very frightening for many men, physicians or not. Talking about them can be very helpful and can give perspective. Only a small percentage of these men are actually homosexual, trapped in marriage, and at some stage of "coming out." In many men, the homosexual concern is a symptom of something underlying that is the real issue and which requires assessment and treatment. Some examples are an undiagnosed depression or obsessional disorder; problems with masculine self-esteem and self-confidence; post-traumatic sequelae of having been sexually assaulted earlier in life; abuse of drugs that are disinhibiting; marital problems characterized by unassertiveness and ruminating; and other life stresses that are affecting the physician's sense of mastery, power, independence, and control.[40]

Dr. and Mrs. W were a young couple in their late twenties when they came for marital therapy. Mrs. W was seven months pregnant. When I asked them to tell me about their concerns, Mrs. W started to cry, reached for some tissue paper, and told her husband to start. His face ashen, Dr. W stated, "I guess I'm gay." With this, he began to cry, too.

Dr. W said that he had been finding himself having a lot of thoughts and sexual feelings about other men for the past three months. They were with him whenever he was not at work or otherwise engaged in some activity. He was both curious and frightened about this. Although he had never had a homosexual experience, he had wondered from time to time since he was a teenager if he might be gay. He had been tempted to go to a gay bar or to pick up a male prostitute "just to find out." He and Mrs. W were very open about all of this; she was devastated but sympathetic to his inner confusion and unhappiness.

I completed a very thorough assessment of Dr. W over the course of this conjoint visit and two visits with him alone. He was not gay. He was suffering from an obsessional disorder with intrusive and repetitive homosexual thoughts of oral and anal sex. In public he found himself "checking out men's penises and buns." This disturbed him so much that he had become reluctant to go downtown alone. He was afraid that he might make a pass at a stranger.

Dr. W was also clinically depressed (he had lost fifteen pounds, he was awakening at four a.m. every day, he had trouble concentrating on his medical work, he had intermittent thoughts of suicide, and his energy level was greatly reduced). Furthermore, he had never had any interest in kissing, holding hands with, hugging, being in love with, being emotionally intimate with, or being in a committed relationship with a man. In fact, he was quite repelled by many of my questions about nonsexual or loving matters between men!

His thoughts were totally erotic and genital. And they were wearing him down. I explained to him, and to his wife, my diagnostic impression and my thoughts about treatment. She was reassured; he was not. His wariness and lack of confidence about my diagnosis and plan were a further manifestation of his depression. In short, he was quite convinced that he was gay—which meant to him that he was second-class, perverted, sick, a burden to his wife, and a lousy husband and father-to-be. His guilt was terrible.

Fortunately, he was agreeable to a second opinion by a highly respected and openly gay psychiatrist in our medical community. This man agreed with my diagnosis. With this, Dr. W agreed to accept antidepressant and anti-obsessional medication and supportive psychotherapy from me. He also began to do some reading that I suggested on cognitive therapy, with a number of recommended self-help exercises. Over the next three to four weeks, his obsessive thoughts about gay sex and men's anatomy lessened and ended. His mood improved. He became involved once again in the excitement of having a baby and became more secure with his heterosexuality.

Because this can be a very complex and confusing problem, not only for the physician-patient but also for his wife, it is imperative that sound professional help be obtained. Serious consequences for the health of the doctor and his marriage can result from hasty, ill-advised, or completely erroneous statements by the therapist. Any physician struggling with issues like these who does not feel comfortable with the professional help he is getting should definitely obtain a second opinion. Another opinion is especially important if the situation is worsening rapidly. In general, a combined approach of individual and conjoint therapy is indicated.

VIOLENCE

Violence has become epidemic in North American families, and doctors' families are not immune. Physicians' abuse of their wives ranges from the man who has struck his wife once and is now in therapy to understand and control his physical aggression to the man who is a classic wife-beater, that is, a mildly remorseful, easily threatened, impulsive, and controlling man whose assaults are repetitive. Generally, men in this latter group are not amenable to treatment unless their wives have already left, charges have been laid, and the treatment is court ordered.

Most marital therapists are accustomed to working with couples in whose relationship violence has been a concern. In general, only the milder end of the spectrum is responsive to couple therapy—where both individuals are deeply upset and want to do something about it. The couple and the therapist must agree on basic principles: Male domination by physical force is wrong, immoral, and contrary to egalitarian partnership in marriage; there is never any justification for or defense of hitting or physical coercion in marriage; and essentially, violence in marriage means men battering women. The argument that some women in marriages are violent and beat their husbands is largely spurious. Women who strike their husbands are usually doing so in self-defense, but there are indeed some women with very poor impulse control who strike out physically when arguing. And they strike out first and perhaps solely (i.e., their husbands do not strike back). I have never seen a seriously battered husband. I wish the opposite were true.

Mrs. E was a thirty-four-year-old woman who came to see me from a safe house, a shelter for battered women. She had fled her husband one week earlier after a beating. After receiving treatment at a local emergency room for bruises, abrasions, and a broken wrist, she charged her husband with assault and began counseling sponsored by an antiviolence support group. Her husband was arrested and spent a night in jail. He was then ordered by the courts to pay a fine and to enter group treatment for assaultive men.

Mrs. E's husband was a surgeon; she was a bank manager. They had been married for five years and had no children. Both had come from verbally and physically abusive backgrounds. There was a lot of alcoholism in each of their families—and Dr. E drank a lot, especially on weekends. Dr. E first beat his wife about six months into their relationship, just after they began living together. The precipitant was that she had not shined his shoes to his liking (he was extremely domineering, controlling, and sadistic in his attitude toward her). What followed were years of cyclical and repeated assaults and harmonious periods, with progressive erosion of Mrs. E's self-esteem, confidence, and assertiveness. She shared her shameful secret with no one except a sister in Southeast Asia.

Dr. and Mrs. E remained separated for eighteen months. During that time, Dr. E completed group therapy and learned new ways of communicating. He also became involved in AA and IDAA (International Doctors in AA). Both of them became born-again Christians and found great comfort and fellowship in their church and minister. My work with Mrs. E was largely supportive and cautionary. She benefited tremendously from group therapy with other victims of violence—and from Alanon. I only had a few conjoint visits with the two of them when they began dating each other again and after they reconciled.

In a situation in which the doctor has struck his wife in response to interpersonal tension, marital treatment can be helpful. It is sometimes possible to identify antecedent statements or feelings that arise just prior to the physical outburst. Is he lashing out in self-defense? Is he feeling put down, frightened, insulted, or impotent? Does he feel verbally inept compared to his wife? Or is he feeling resentful, spiteful, or vindictive from previous marital upsets and hurts? Is there an underlying substrate of unresolved rage and hatred toward his wife so that minimal activity on her part leads to extreme physical aggression on his part? Is he disinhibited by excessive use of alcohol or drugs? Answers to these questions may be illuminating and pave the way toward more effective and nonviolent forms of communication in the marriage.

SYMPTOMATIC CHILD AS IDENTIFIED PATIENT

Some doctors and their wives have no conscious awareness of a marital problem. Their main concern is anxiety and frustration with a psychiatrically ill child. Their son or daughter may be having behavioral difficulties in school (e.g., aggressive outbursts, stealing, truancy), phobic symptoms, various types of physical symptoms, an eating disorder, or persistent slipping of grades. Some physicians or their wives are aware of marital unhappiness and tension but have not understood its impact on the health of their children until they (the children) become quite symptomatic.

An example of this type of situation occurred with Dr. and Mrs. A, who came for marital therapy because they were worried about their twelve-year-old son, Alex. They had had marital troubles for many years but never sought therapy. They told me that over the previous six months, Alex had really changed—he was fighting with both of them, was constantly on the defensive, refused to tell them where he was going when he went out, and had slipped the past semester from being a solid B student to barely passing. He had come home "either drunk or stoned" on a couple of occasions, and he had been hard to arouse several mornings for school. His parents were also worried about the kids he was hanging around with, a very different group from the year before.

Assessment by a child psychiatrist is the first step in treatment. He or she will be able to tease out the various contributing factors (the parents' marriage, each parent's relationship with the child and vice versa, the child's intrinsic temperament, sibling interactions, and extrafamilial influences) and map out with the doctor and his wife the most appropriate and efficient therapeutic approaches. I will have more to say about the specifics of treatment in Chapter Eight.

CONCLUSION

I have briefly outlined some of the worries with which doctors and/or their wives contend. This is a taste, a sampling only, of a far-reaching range of concerns in doctors' marriages. Much has been written elsewhere about the most common afflictions in doctors: job stress,[41-44] alcoholism,[9,19-22] drug abuse,[20-25,27-31] and depression.[27,33,45] I have concentrated only on the relationship of these illnesses to marriage. Many of these marital concerns are not specific to male doctors; many are seen in the marriages of men in other professions. Some are seen in the marriages of women doctors, as will be discussed in the next chapter.

These problem areas have been observed in those medical couples who come to see a psychiatrist. There are undoubtedly many other anxieties, both specific and thematic, with which doctors and their wives struggle, anxieties that have never been aired and have escaped clinical scrutiny and empirical study. Those unique to medical marriages are most important; as they are discovered, we will have a clearer understanding of causation, means of prevention, and therapeutic intervention.

REFERENCES

1. Michael Garvey and Vicente B. Tuason, "Physician Marriages," *Journal of Clinical Psychiatry* 40 (1979), 129–131.
2. S. E. D. Shortt, "Psychiatric Illness in Physicians," *Canadian Medical Association Journal* 121 (1979), 283–288.
3. Robert Krell and James E. Miles, "Marital Therapy of Couples in Which the Husband Is a Physician," *American Journal of Psychotherapy* 30 (1976), 267–275.
4. Martin Goldberg, "Conjoint Therapy of Male Physicians and Their Wives," *Psychiatric Opinion* 12 (1975), 19–23.
5. Edward M. Waring, "Psychiatric Illness in Physicians: A Review," *Comprehensive Psychiatry* 15 (1974), 519–530.
6. Carla Fine, *Married to Medicine* (New York: Atheneum, 1981).
7. J. K. Skipper, Jr., and W. A. Gliebe, "Forgotten Persons: Physicians' Wives and Their Influence on Medical Career Decisions," *Journal of Medical Education* 52 (1977), 764–766.
8. James E. Miles, Robert Krell, and Tsung Y. Li, "The Doctor's Wife: Mental Illness and Marital Pattern," *International Journal of Psychiatry in Medicine* 6 (1975), 481–487.
9. M. M. Pearson, "Psychiatric Treatment of 250 Physicians," *Psychiatric Annals* 12 (1982), 194–206.
10. Lane A. Gerber, *Married to Their Careers: Career and Family Dilemmas in Doctors' Lives* (New York: Tavistock, 1983).
11. Glen O. Gabbard and Roy W. Menninger, *Medical Marriages* (Washington, D.C.: American Psychiatric Press, 1988).
12. Esther Nitzberg, *Hippocrates' Handmaidens: Women Married to Physicians* (New York: Haworth, 1991).

13. Clifford J. Sager, *Marriage Contracts and Couple Therapy* (New York: Brunner/Mazel, 1976), 19–20.
14. Deborah Tannen, *You Just Don't Understand: Women and Men in Conversation* (New York: Ballantine, 1990), 17–18.
15. Glen O. Gabbard, "The Role of Compulsiveness in the Normal Physician," *Journal of the American Medical Association* 254 (1985), 2926–2929.
16. Joanna Jones Ellis and Donald R. Inbody, "Psychotherapy With Physicians' Families: When Attributes in Medical Practice Become Liabilities in Family Life," *American Journal of Psychotherapy* 42 (July 1988), 380–388.
17. Peter A. Martin and H. W. Bird, "The 'Love-Sick' Wife and the 'Cold-Sick' Husband," *Psychiatry* 22 (1959), 245–249.
18. Barbara Killinger, *Workaholics: The Respectable Addicts. A Family Survival Guide* (Toronto: Key Porter Books, 1991).
19. Leclair Bissell and Robert W. Jones, "The Alcoholic Physician: A Survey," *American Journal of Psychiatry* 133 (1976), 1142–1146.
20. Thomas G. Webster, "Problems of Drug Addiction and Alcoholism Among Physicians," in *The Impaired Physician,* ed. Stephen C. Scheiber and Brian B. Doyle (New York: Plenum Press, 1983), 27–38.
21. George E. Vaillant, Jane R. Brighton, and Charles McArthur, "Physicians' Use of Mood-Altering Drugs," *New England Journal of Medicine* 282 (February 12, 1970), 365–370.
22. Group for the Advancement of Psychiatry, Committee on Alcoholism and the Addictions, "Substance Abuse Disorders: A Psychiatric Priority," *American Journal of Psychiatry* 148 (October 1991), 1291–1300.
23. "Doctors Helping Doctors: Concerned Physicians Step Out in Vanguard Georgia Program," *Alcoholism* 1 (1981), 25–27.
24. Douglas A. Sargent, "The Impaired Physician Movement: An Interim Report," *Hospital and Community Psychiatry* 36 (March 1985), 294–297.
25. Marc Galanter, Douglas Talbott, Karl Gallegos, and Elizabeth Rubenstone, "Combined Alcoholics Anonymous and Professional Care for Addicted Physicians," *American Journal of Psychiatry* 147 (January 1990), 64–68.
26. Michael F. Myers, "Fighting Stigma: How to Help the Doctor's Family," in *Stigma and Mental Illness,* ed. Paul J. Fink and Allan Tasman (Washington, D.C.: American Psychiatric Press, 1992), 140.
27. Robert E. Jones, "A Study of 100 Physician Psychiatric Inpatients," *American Journal of Psychiatry* 134 (1977), 1119–1123.
28. R. P. Johnson and J. C. Connelly, "Addicted Physicians: A Closer Look," *Journal of the American Medical Association* 245 (1981), 253–257.
29. H. Wallott and J. Lambert, "Characteristics of Physician Addicts," *American Journal of Drug and Alcohol Abuse* 10 (1984), 53–62.
30. William E. McAuliffe, Mary Rohman, Susan Santangelo, Barry Feldman, Elizabeth Magnuson, Arthur Sobol, and Joel Weissman, "Psychoactive Drug Use Among Practicing Physicians and Medical Students," *New England Journal of Medicine* 315 (September 25, 1986), 805–810.
31. George E. Vaillant, "Physician, Cherish Thyself: The Hazards of Self-Prescribing," *Journal of the American Medical Association* 267 (May 6, 1992), 2373–2374.
32. George E. Vaillant, N. C. Sobowale, and C. McArthur, "Some Psychologic Vulnerabilities of Physicians," *New England Journal of Medicine* 287 (1972), 372–375.
33. "Depression: Having It Made Me See It," *Minnesota Medicine* 74 (August 1991), 13.
34. John La Puma, Carl B. Stocking, Dan La Voie, and Cheryl A. Darling, "When Physi-

cians Treat Members of Their Own Families," *New England Journal of Medicine* 325 (October 31, 1991), 1290–1294.

35. Alan A. Stone, "Sexual Exploitation of Patients in Psychotherapy," in *Law, Psychiatry, and Morality,* ed. Alan A. Stone (Washington, D.C.: American Psychiatric Press, 1984), 191–216.

36. Nanette Gartrell, Judith Herman, Silvia Olarte, Michael Feldstein, and Russell Localio, "Psychiatrist–Patient Sexual Contact, Results of a National Survey: I. Prevalence," *American Journal of Psychiatry* 143 (September 1986), 1126–1131.

37. Glen O. Gabbard, *Sexual Exploitation in Professional Relationships* (Washington, D.C.: American Psychiatric Press, 1989).

38. Council on Ethical and Judicial Affairs, American Medical Association, "Sexual Misconduct in the Practice of Medicine," *Journal of the American Medical Association* 266 (November 20, 1991), 2741–2745.

39. Stella L. Blackshaw and Paul G. R. Patterson, "The Prevention of Sexual Exploitation of Patients: Educational Issues," *Canadian Journal of Psychiatry* 37 (June 1992), 350–353.

40. Richard C. Friedman, *Male Homosexuality: A Contemporary Psychoanalytic Perspective* (New Haven, Conn.: Yale University Press, 1988).

41. Ronald J. Burke and Astrid M. Richardsen, "Sources of Satisfaction and Stress Among Canadian Physicians," *Psychological Reports* 67 (1990), 1335–1344.

42. Timothy E. Quill and Penelope R. Williamson, "Healthy Approaches to Physician Stress," *Archives of Internal Medicine* 150 (September 1990), 1857–1861.

43. Layne A. Simpson and Linda Grant, "Sources and Magnitude of Job Stress Among Physicians," *Journal of Behavioral Medicine* 14 (1991), 27–42.

44. Michael E. Gallery, Theodore W. Whitley, Leah K. Klonis, Robert K. Anzinger, and Dennis A. Revicki, "A Study of Occupational Stress and Depression Among Emergency Physicians," *Annals of Emergency Medicine* 21 (January 1992), 58–64.

45. T. E. Bittker, "Reaching Out to the Depressed Physician," *Journal of the American Medical Association* 236 (1976), 1713–1716.

Chapter Three

FEMALE PHYSICIAN MARRIAGES

Although women doctors were a thriving and vocal group in the late nineteenth century, we do not know a lot about their personal lives and, in particular, their marriages. Indeed, many did not marry, tending instead to devote all of their time, energy, and nurturance to their patients and community service. In this century, and until the early 1970s, the numbers of women in medicine were very small; women doctors were excluded from virtually all in-depth studies of medical students, housestaff, office practice, and academic medicine.[1] Publications on medical marriages focused entirely on male physicians and doctors' wives.

Since the early 1970s, quotas have been lifted and approximately 40% of medical students today are women. There is now a significant body of scholarship on the unique and gender-specific concerns of women who are doctors, and this work includes research on their marriages.[2–11]

I would like now to delineate the more common marital problems of women doctors who request professional help. Although I have published some of these findings previously,[12–14] I want to update and expand upon some of them as well as describe newer considerations. These findings are a mix of direct observation and subjectively reported feelings and symptoms.

DELAY IN SEEKING HELP

Delay in seeking help is not unique to the marriages of women doctors—male physicians especially delay getting help, as do couples in general. The reasons for this hesitation or resistance vary from couple to couple, but there are several: Multiple commitments to work, children, running the home, extended family, and community preclude time for one's marriage and marital therapy; there is often denial of the seriousness of marital unhappiness and estrangement until a crisis occurs;

75

pride in one's reserve and ability to cope with stress and personal adversity militates against reaching out for assistance; embarrassment and guilt about "having problems" frequently accompanies the perfectionism of many doctors; complete unavailability of appropriate treatment resources in the community, especially in smaller and rural settings, reinforces resistance to therapy; and relative lack of specialized treatment, that is, where privacy and confidentiality can be ensured, where conflicts of interest between therapist and doctor-patient do not occur, and where therapists who are skilled in marital work with women doctors are in practice. Historically, it has always been difficult for doctors with personal problems to ask for help, and it still is for older physicians. It is refreshing that medical students and residents come forward much more easily now than was the case a generation ago.

Like many other contemporary women, some female physicians have had an earlier experience with a male therapist that was negative; this colors one's attitude toward future help tremendously, but most female physicians will accept a female therapist. They anticipate, usually correctly, that another woman professional will have both an intellectual and experiential sensitivity to the stresses of balancing career and marriage. Many doctors prefer a nonpsychiatrist for marital treatment: They do not have to worry about being given a psychiatric label; they will get counseling and not merely drugs; their experience with psychiatrists as consultants and colleagues has been less than winsome; and they harbor feelings of failure and demoralization about their marriages and feel ashamed to disclose to another medical person.

Let me give an example of a woman doctor, Dr. W, who had had nothing but bad experiences with the male psychiatrists whom she had consulted in the past. I saw her with her husband and she opened the visit with, "I want to be very frank with you. I'm not sure if this is going to work, that is, our seeing a male doctor for our marriage. Quite apart from the fact that our marriage is in trouble and we need help, I'm only here because you are specialized in doctors' marriages and because Tom said he'd rather see a man, than a woman." After Dr. W and Mr. G, her husband, told me about their marital worries and problems, I asked Dr. W to tell me a bit more about their previous therapy experiences.

They first saw a psychiatrist toward the end of Dr. W's internship year. "I was seven months pregnant, and Tom and I were fighting a lot. Probably because of a combination of factors—we hardly knew each other, we had only met a year earlier, we had money worries, and I was tired and irritable a lot of the time." Mr. G added, "And I couldn't find a steady job, which got me down; I was really worried about the responsibility of becoming a father." Dr. W continued, "So we went to see Dr. A, who was recommended by my train-ing director. He was terrible. He cut us off in the middle of our first visit and proceeded to lecture me about women in medicine trying to do it all and driving themselves and others around them nuts. He chastised me for my plans to start my residency and to get a nanny. He also told me that in his clini-cal experience, most husbands of residents 'fool around' and that I should think seriously about that. Tom almost punched him. Needless to say, we never went back."

Dr. W then proceeded to tell me about a more recent experience they had had with a male psychiatrist, Dr. N. "Things started out OK. About the third or fourth visit, Tom and I were talking about a fight we had had the day before and things got pretty heated in the office. Dr. N turned to me and said, 'You do get quite hostile, don't you? I can understand now why you [turning to Tom] withdraw like you do.' I was furious and told him I resented his remark. I really didn't want to go back the following week but decided I would and that I would bring up the incident for discussion. I did. I told him I felt hurt . . . and picked on . . . and singled out. What infuriated me, again, was his response to me, which was so patronizing, so stereotypically psychiatric, something like, 'Ac-cepting the truths about ourselves is one of the hardest facets of psychotherapy.' I kept my mouth shut and refused to go back to him."

Dr. W had had a much earlier negative experience with a male psychiatrist whom she saw when she was a medical student. She had become depressed after she and her boyfriend broke up and her grades began to fall. The psychiatrist insisted she take an antidepressant medication, despite her strong reluctance to do so. "He just wouldn't listen to me. I told him I wasn't that depressed, that I just needed to talk and be listened to and reassured, that I'd be OK, and get better again. He said we could do both. So I took the pills. He still didn't listen. He just asked about side effects and changed the subject when I tried to speak about my feelings."

In most couples, it is the woman who first suggests and who initiates marital help. Most men balk at the idea first time around, and in some cases, many times around. Weeks, months, or years may pass before husbands consent to treatment. I have talked with many women doctors who came to the realization of the need for outside intervention a long time before the first visit with me, but their husbands steadfastly refused to begin therapy. For some of these women nothing short of threatening divorce unless help is obtained has worked.

The resistance of men to therapy has multiple determinants: a need to be strong, capable, and self-reliant; blatant denial of any marital problem; fear of the unknown, that is, therapy; feelings of embarrass-ment (this may be more pronounced in husbands who are physicians themselves); an intense sense of privacy regarding personal and marital matters; fears of being "one down" in a verbal or psychologically oriented milieu that is considered more a woman's domain; or a previous therapy experience that was negative (e.g., nothing happened, the therapist was cool or distant, husband felt blamed).[15-16] As one can see, these are very significant and very valid reasons to delay or avoid seeking help altogether.

GUILT

The feeling of guilt is always present in women doctors with marital trouble. Usually, this tendency to blame oneself is part of the woman doctor's personality; in other words, she is self-blaming in many other aspects of her life as well. It is a component of perfectionism and is felt and expressed when the woman cannot live up to the expectations of herself. Superwomen, and their aspirants, to use the vernacular of the 1980s, know this emotion all too well. In the 1990s, it is my impression that women in the professions are striving less to be "superwoman" and accepting that they cannot do it all (and feeling better for it).

I am not talking about the usual and ever-present feelings of guilt that most people have who are concerned about their marriages. I mean something more than this. I am talking about the woman doctor who breaks out in anxiety and depressive symptoms and who is not able to implicate external forces in their causation. For example, her husband may be drinking excessively, her secretary may be less than competent, and her daughter may be rebelling at home, yet she reacts to all of these problems by feeling like a failure. She berates herself for being disorganized and tells herself she just needs to try harder. Some women physicians who feel like this have underlying problems with their self-esteem and struggle with feelings of inadequacy, which tend to compound a guilty nature. And if they are somewhat isolated from other professional women who are trying to cope with this life-balancing dilemma, they may not realize that many of their feelings are normal.

The problem of guilt may be reinforced if the woman physician is treated only for the symptoms, that is, with medication, and none of the intrapsychic and interpersonal marital and family dynamics are explored. I will elaborate on this later when I talk about treatment. It is also critical that a serious clinical depression not be missed, one of the hallmarks of which is guilt. This must be distinguished from what I have said above.

When Dr. Y sat down in my office for her first visit, her opening words were: "Thank you for taking the time to see me. You are a very busy man, and I'll try to only bother you for this one visit. My best friend is Dr. M [a work acquaintance of mine], and he insisted that I see you. I feel so guilty. I've already been to see Dr. P. She says I'm depressed and gave me a prescription for an antidepressant. I'm supposed to see her tomorrow, and I haven't even filled the prescription! I'm not sure if I'm depressed. I hate the idea of taking medicine. I told her that and she said to just follow her advice and in three weeks I'll feel much much better. Maybe I should go now. This isn't right, going from one psychiatrist to another. I'm wasting your time."

Dr. Y's statements spoke volumes. In that first visit I learned that she wasn't clinically depressed, but she certainly was worn down from an enormous number of responsibilities in her life. She was a single parent, and her estranged husband had contributed nothing to the expenses of raising two young daughters. She had a very busy and successful practice in family medicine. Dr. Y often worked late and did extra call, not because of money worries, but because she felt guilty saying no to literally everyone.

What was interesting, and not known to Dr. Y, is that her parents had been patients of mine some years earlier. They were having marital problems after the death of Dr. Y's sister from toxic shock syndrome. I remembered them as a gracious couple who were very likeable, talented, and community-involved individuals. When I reviewed their file, I saw that I had noted in the margin, "These two both are perpetually guilty!" So Dr. Y came by her guilt quite naturally.

Dr. Y did well in short-term therapy. What helped her the most is an assertiveness training group for women in medicine that I recommended she consider attending.

SELF-IMAGE PROBLEMS

Those doctors who are not confident about themselves as women will have a lot of difficulty feeling secure in their marriages. This insecurity is more prevalent in the early years of marriage before a good level of honest communication and complete trust has been established. Later in the marriage, both the woman and her husband will have identified, disclosed, discussed, and accepted their mutual areas of vulnerability and insecurity—it is hoped. But for many couples this fundamental work of marriage just doesn't get done. Only the day-to-day issues and the "nice stuff" are talked about. For many it takes a crisis to begin to get at that deeper, and more frightening, level of communication.

The woman doctor who is unsure of herself as a woman will feel one down in marriage. Even if she doesn't feel one down, she acts as one who is down. She will not be comfortably asserting herself and challenging her husband, she will quiver at his control and domination, she will fear he will be unfaithful, or she will be rendered powerless by his flirtations with other women. She will fear abandonment. In sum, she is tremendously disadvantaged.

Some women who study medicine have not grown up with a comfortable and consolidated sense of themselves as being appealing or attractive. For some women, their scholastic achievement and ambition alone set them apart from peers of both sexes and contribute to this subjective sense of unattractiveness. This feeling is especially so for women who are raised in homes and communities with norms and values that are quite traditional or rigid, where bright and striving women are seen as deviant or as an oddity. Sociocultural forces like these profoundly influence one's developing sexual and personal identity, with far-reaching consequences. Once in medical school, these same women may be subjected to similar influential forces.

Let me explain. Until the 1970s, women in medicine, for the most part, were stereotyped and largely misunderstood. Because they had entered a predominantly male profession, many were perceived and judged as "masculine" regardless of appearance. Others were seen as "sexless." Many were simply ignored. Those women who actually fit or fulfilled the male social definition of female attractiveness or desirability were suspect, that is, their appearance was seen as "just a front" or if not a front, perhaps a sign that they weren't that bright or serious about medicine after all. They were derided for being in medical school for their "Mrs.," not their "M.D." Heaven help the female medical student who was in essence quite sexy, for she really was in a no-win situation—adored one minute, ogled the next, and ultimately rejected as "inappropriately dressed for a doctor" or "sleeping her way through medical school."

This was an epoch in medicine before the study of gender and gender roles in the academic setting and workplace. Women medical students were not asked to identify or talk about their feelings while dissecting male genitalia in anatomy classes, or while examining male patients on the wards. There was no discussion or teaching about what to do when a patient gets an erection, or how to handle sexist (was there such a word then?) jokes and male doctors who called their female patients "honey." Women students did not know what to do when certain professors and clinical supervisors touched or rubbed against them in ways that did not feel quite right. Furthermore, they did not know what to call this harassment; inevitably, they tried to dismiss it or blamed themselves for their discomfort. There was no one with whom to talk about these things.

I will not belabor this. My point is that when a doctor struggles with her self-image as a woman, it is not just a genetic predisposition, or that her mother had the same problem, or that her father was absent or aloof. It is a complex mix of biopsychosocial factors. When she can understand this, and when her husband understands and appreciates this as well, then there will be much less tension, less confusion, and more equitable balance of power in the relationship.

IMPAIRED ASSERTIVENESS IN MARITAL COMMUNICATION

For some women doctors there is an incongruity between their assertiveness at work and their assertiveness in marriage. These women are clear and straightforward with their patients, their students, and other physicians and staff, but quite different with their husbands. They may have difficulty identifying their needs and complaints as legitimate and when they do, they have difficulty articulating them directly and with conviction. There may be several reasons for this: a general sense of unworthiness and inadequacy in relationships with men, another aspect of the self-image problems mentioned above; a low-grade generalized depression that alters one's sense of self and assertiveness in personal functioning but spares professional functioning; an inordinate need to do all of the traditionally female household work oneself with a poor capacity for delegating tasks and responsibility; and a husband who is unapproachable, controlling, intimidating, and perhaps violent.

Many contemporary women physicians have difficulty with sex-role change, reversal, and fluidity. Most, and their husbands, have come from traditional backgrounds: Their mothers did everything in the home, and their fathers did everything outside. These "scripts" are powerful and deeply ingrained. Becoming more assertive about sharing child care and domestic chores in marriage requires experimentation, negotiation, and practice. Statements like, "I still feel guilty every time my husband irons his shirts," or "There's something about my husband's cleaning toilets that bothers me," despite the humor, are not uncommon.

I am struck by the attitude of protectiveness and defensiveness toward their husbands that I witness in some of my women physician patients. On the surface, this is quite lovely, this sense of respectfulness, caring, and sensitivity. But in some cases, there are ramifications. They may be paying a price by their manner and stance, and quite a price at that. They may be unwittingly subordinating their own needs to those of their husbands. They are being shortchanged, and they don't even know it. In some cases, defensiveness about their husbands' shortcomings and liabilities is coupled with resentment and unhappiness.

This type of marital dynamic is most apt to occur when two factors are present: first, the woman physician herself does not have a healthy sense of self-worth but covers it well, and second, her husband denies that he has problems and will not seek help for them. Her defensiveness will be sparked when friends and family withdraw from her husband and criticize her for remaining with him. Several examples come to mind: the woman physician whose husband is alcoholic and refuses treatment; the woman physician who is ashamed to tell anyone that her husband beats her; the woman whose husband is repeatedly unfaithful; the woman whose husband is chronically out of work and whom she supports; the woman whose husband has a well-compensated paranoid character and who subtly and cleverly diminishes her as the years go by; and the woman whose husband is antisocial, always in debt, and expects to be bailed out.

Often people ask, "Why do women remain in marriages like these?" They remain for many reasons. The most common is to preserve a sense of family when there are young children. Many married individuals dread the idea of their children experiencing a marital breakup and try to avoid it if at all possible. Many men categorically refuse to accept marital help, so their physician wives feel paralyzed. Some women in medicine are very caretaking, and this extends into their marriages. Many people fear being alone, and they associate separation with aloneness. Others remain eternally hopeful that things might improve "down the road." And there continues to be at least some stigma associated with divorce, and this preys on unhappily married women who do not feel strong enough to cope with it.

I want to conclude this section by mentioning the pivotal research of Carol Gilligan.[17] In her book *In a Different Voice: Psychological Theory and Women's Development*, Gilligan describes how women define themselves in terms of relationships to others, in terms of the care of others, by taking responsibility in relationships, and by responsive engagement. Her observations are germane to an understanding of women doctors, whose marriages I have discussed earlier. Gilligan's ideas help to explain these marriages and place the woman in a value-free context, that is, one in which she is not accused of being stupid, masochistic, or a martyr. Her behavior in marriage is gender defined, part of being female in Western culture, and not necessarily a deep-seated or intrapsychic problem. With these insights, the woman can more clearly see what is happening and begin to work toward change, including separation and divorce if necessary.

ROLE STRAIN

Role strain refers to the difficulty and frustration in trying to meet the demands of many roles. For married women doctors with children these demands include their roles as physicians, wives, mothers, and usually executive managers of their homes. When women doctors are not meeting these obligations as well as they would like, or feel they should be, they may become symptomatic. A typical picture includes anxiety, panic attacks, guilt, forgetfulness, insomnia, self-castigation, irritability, and loss of their characteristic and highly developed organizing ability. Needless to say, these feelings usually spill over into the marriage, homeostasis is upset, and marital conflict ensues.

Role strain can be both a cause and a result of marital difficulty. Situations in which men are not assisting at home with the children, marketing, chores, and so forth, or are not doing their fair share, are a breeding ground for role strain as the women already overburdened try to take on more. If the woman and her husband are fighting or not getting along, he may be withdrawn and not helping out as much as usual, or he may be going out more to avoid being home and in this way relinquishing his paternal and household responsibilities. Women who try to do too much themselves, who do not assign jobs easily, and whose husbands are not perceptive, not forthcoming, sexist, or just plain lazy are prime candidates for role strain.

Role strain leads to marital difficulty when the woman doctor cannot stand it anymore. She finds herself angry and resentful. Her husband, in turn, grows weary of her fatigue and yelling; he feels picked on, put down, and unappreciated. He counterattacks with his own put-downs or starts making inappropriate and unsolicited suggestions, urging her to quit working or to hire a second nanny for weekends. These serve only to fuel the fire. Both partners continue to feel angry, hurt, and misunderstood.

Many husbands of doctors suffer from role strain, too, but do not always articulate it as such. They are trying to fulfill the demands of their jobs as well as attempting to be more attentive and more involved husbands and fathers than they perceived their own fathers to be. Most of these men are in a professional field themselves, and their work is not just a job but a career. Many feel torn because they are at a stage of their careers that requires a lot of time investment, evening and weekend work, and sometimes travel. This stage corresponds with the time in their personal lives when their children are young, growing and changing rapidly, and needy. Some try to do their best to balance the needs of their wives and children with their work, some opt for the "fast track," and others yield to the pull of their domestic and nurturing side. Unfortunately, many employers, organizations, and institutions are not that "male-gender friendly" (i.e., they are not very sensitive to or supportive of men who wish to work a reduced schedule, or share a position, or have paternity leave, or take some other measure in order to have more time with their families).

In many female physician marriages that I have seen, both partners are overstressed. In essence, they are trying to do too much as individuals and as couples. It is truly remarkable what they accomplish in a week and how well organized they are in coordinating everything. They meet career demands, work-related commitments, household responsibilities, social obligations, and the needs of their respective extended families. They spend weekends running errands and being with their children. But what they don't do is budget or schedule time just for the two of them, for talk, relaxation, sex, and entertainment. This budgeting is essential. Their lives are too hectic and fast paced; without time for themselves, daily tensions spill into the marriage, misinterpretations set in, and gradual erosion of marital intimacy can develop.

Here is a not-uncommon example of role strain in a physician's marriage:

Dr. White and her husband, Mr. Smith, came to their first appointment with this as their chief complaint: "We've decided to separate, unless you're a miracle worker or something. Our marriage is dead, we can barely tolerate each other, and now we're both so stressed we're getting sick." I asked for more details.

Dr. White was forty years old and a family practitioner in a group practice in a medium-sized city in British Columbia. Mr. Smith was forty-two years old and an accountant. They had been married for ten years and had three children (eight, six, and three years old). Both felt that their marital relationship had changed dramatically since their youngest child was born. They had not been out together as a couple in over a year; they felt like they were ships passing in the night. They were often tense with each other, bickered a lot, had days of stony silence, and from time to time slept in separate rooms because "he snores." Mr. Smith admitted that he was drinking more than usual; Dr. White admitted she had been taking Ativan from her samples at work to sleep at night for more than two years. They had not made love in about eighteen months.

When I tried to assess their level of busyness, here is what I was told:

Dr. White worked four days a week in her office, did all her own deliveries (about six per month), assisted in the operating room when her patients were in surgery, volunteered once a week at a local foodbank, served on two hospital committees, coached her daughter's field hockey team, attended virtually all of her kids' athletic events, supervised their homework and music practice, attended Bible study one evening per week and church every Sunday, taught Sunday school every other week, and was in the middle of writing a whole-earth cookbook. Mr. Smith was a principal in his firm, traveled at least once a week to Vancouver on business, was active in the Rotary Club (and was on the executive committee), played old-boys' rugby and hockey, coached his son's baseball team, was renovating the basement to build a recreation room for the kids, and was in the midst of launching a provincewide data system for continuing education for chartered accountants. He was also grieving the loss of his parents, who tragically had been killed in a car accident three months earlier (in addition to sorting out their estate and contested wills).

HUSBANDS WITH UNMET NEEDS

Husbands of women doctors are an understudied group of men. The majority of women doctors marry other professionals, and it is estimated that from 50% to 70% of these men are doctors themselves. To my knowledge, there has been no systematic examination of these men except for an Australian study of female physicians' perceptions of their husbands (not of the husbands themselves).[18] The personalities, needs and expectations in marriage, values, attitudes toward women, and response patterns to stress of doctors' husbands are largely unknown. How they are similar to and different from professional men who marry women not involved in a career is also unknown. More research is needed on at least three groups of men: (1) a sample of nonmedical husbands, (2) husbands of a maritally distressed group of women physicians, and (3) former husbands of divorced women physicians.

Happily married women doctors credit their husbands' respect and admiration for them as fundamental to marital harmony. Doctors' husbands are distinguished by their maturity, flexibility, and comfort with gender-role change and, at times, reversal (that is, because of unemployment or underemployment in their fields, some doctors' husbands are home full-time as fathers and homemakers).

What about husbands who are not as happily married? What are their concerns, worries, and complaints? In my own study of sixteen female doctors with dysfunctional marriages, twelve of their husbands were troubled with and unhappy about several needs.[19] They com-

plained of not feeling identified and recognized as important to their wives; they felt that they were low on the list of priorities. Some felt unnurtured and in need of attention and care. One man stated, "I just want to be fussed over once in a while." Several did not feel affirmed as men, that is, as workers, good husbands, and good fathers. Some wanted more companionship and friendship with their wives. Some resented the patients' demands on their wives' time. This resentment usually occurred only when their wives were on call, delivering babies, or engrossed in research demands. All the husbands longed for a greater measure of intimacy, emotional closeness, and sexual activity.

Let me clarify these points. For many of these men—in fact, for most—these needs were not conscious. The men were not aware of these concerns and disappointments until after psychotherapy. Hence, they were not able to express these matters clearly and directly to their wives. In fact, their behavior toward their wives was largely unpleasant—morose, disgruntled, bitter, and sarcastic. Many of the women complained about this behavior, but their husbands rarely responded directly; they tended to withdraw into themselves. Half of these men were sexually involved, or had been previously involved, outside their marriages at the time of initial consultation.

Dr. F came to see me alone to talk about his marriage. He was an economist in private industry, his wife a cardiologist. Although he told me that he had tremendous respect for his wife, one would never know it by his bitter complaints and anecdotes about their life together. By the end of our first hour together I wondered why he was still with her—and she with him, if his mood and attitude at home were anything like the way he was with me in my office. We agreed to meet again, and I made the suggestion that I might like to meet with his wife at some point. He balked at this and told me that he had not told his wife about his appointment with me. "That'll just give her more ammunition" were his concluding words. In further visits that we had together, I learned that Dr. F was volcanic in his rage—he never let it out except in my office. I listened to example after example of how he felt insulted and betrayed by his wife: at home as a father and husband, and socially with their friends. I confronted him on his martyring stance and "poor me" posturing, which he had no insight into. As he became more assertive at home and defended himself when he needed to, he felt better, and by inference, so did his wife. His sullen and icy silences at home fell off almost completely.

Dr. F also began to discuss his mixed feelings about his wife's feminism. He praised it one moment and condemned it the next. He described his feelings like this: "Basically I'm for women's rights—100%. I shudder when I contemplate the inequities that still exist in our society, and I'm ashamed when I think

about all the ways in which women are dominated and harmed by men. I consider myself a feminist but not a militant feminist, such as I feel Carol is becoming. It's the radical element, the real man-haters, that concerns me." I *inquired more into this because what Dr. F was harboring was a fear of lesbianism, a fear of Carol becoming "one of them." At a more primitive level, he was afraid of being abandoned and of losing her. Exploring these fears was very helpful and reassuring for him.*

Another aspect of the unmet needs of doctors' husbands has to do with unrealistic expectations of their wives. There are some husbands who have only an intellectual understanding of the revolutionary change in sex roles of women and men in contemporary North America. They may espouse enlightened values, but they have underestimated the profound imprinting that took place while they were growing up in very traditional homes. This imprinting shapes their attitudes toward women as wives and mothers. These men may be shocked at their outdated and inappropriate values and ideas as these thoughts emerge during the early years of marriage or at points of stress. For example, one man said to his physician wife during an argument: "Don't I have a right to expect you to iron my shirts?" Once they have a better understanding of their wives and a more accurate appraisal of what is possible, there is less disappointment, less bitterness, and more harmony.

PROBLEMS WITH INTIMACY AND SEXUALITY

I mentioned above that several husbands in my study wanted more intimacy and sexuality in their marriages. Women doctors with distressed marriages also have this concern and, like women in general, their interest in sex includes a desire for quality time together, communication, romance, and nonsexual affection. In some marriages there is plenty of sex but it has become routine, boring, or a chore. When this situation is not discussed and creative solutions are not discovered, it easily leads to resentment in the woman physician.

Dr. H was not unlike a lot of women who find themselves in a "no win" sexual situation with their husbands. Her complaint was, "I've come to hate sex—I get no pleasure from it anymore. I can't believe that I once enjoyed it—more than enjoyed it actually, I was sexually aggressive!" What Dr. H went on to describe was a daily sexual pattern wherein she accommodated her husband's sexual needs. "My husband's impossible to live with if I don't give it to him. Just hearing myself use those words 'give it to him' upsets me, that I've sunk to this. But it's true, I give in to avoid a hassle. If I beg off, he'll either have a temper tantrum or punish me for twenty-four hours by going cold."

To my knowledge there are no particular sexual dysfunctions unique to women doctors and their husbands. When a sexual problem exists for a couple, it may be one of sexual desire, arousal, or orgasm for either or both partners. Disorders of sexual desire are far more common than the other two types and may be due to reasons that range from deep-seated neurotic conflicts to more superficial concerns such as fatigue, performance anxiety, and unexpressed anger. All couples wherein one or both partners complain of loss of sexual desire should have a very thorough sexual and marital assessment before any specific treatment is instituted.

Some women physicians with sexual difficulties have been sexually abused as girls or sexually assaulted as women. And a high percentage of women physicians have also been subject to sexual harassment while medical students or later in their training. Given the well-known sequelae of these kinds of victimization (i.e., shame, self-blame, fearfulness, loss, mistrustfulness, and sexual inhibitions), it is important that these factors be taken into account whenever a woman doctor and her husband are requesting marital therapy.

Concerns about intimacy involve much more than the communication barriers to sharing private thoughts and feelings. When a doctor complains that her marriage lacks intimacy, she is usually talking about many different facets of her relationship with her husband. There may be a decrease in the level of physical affection shown from one to the other. They may be less verbally expressive together, that is, they do not directly vocalize liking and loving each other as they once did. Women in the early years of marriage may feel that they are not as compatible with their husbands as they had believed, that their backgrounds and values are more dissimilar than they originally felt. A woman may sense a loss of intimacy when her relationship with her husband lacks primacy, or she may feel that it is no longer the most important of all her relationships. In this regard, she may no longer feel part of a couple in the context of her relationships with friends, her family, his family, or even their children.

WHEN THE WOMAN PHYSICIAN IS NOT "ALLOWED" TO HAVE EMOTIONAL NEEDS

When Henry Higgins asked his famous rhetorical question "Why can't a woman be more like a man?" in *My Fair Lady*, he must have had husbands of women doctors in mind! Some of these men have a lot of difficulty perceiving and accepting their wives' needs for support. Some also are made very anxious by the range of emotion shown when their wives are upset about something. I say "anxious" despite the fact that they rarely verbalize this feeling directly. Instead, their behaviors toward their wives consist of sarcasm and put-downs; accusations of her "getting hysterical," "making a mountain out of a molehill," or "dramatizing again"; a cool, controlled, and paternalistic manner; unsolicited advice giving and other practical suggestions; emotional withholding; and walking out of the room.

I am aware that I am generalizing here about the gender-specific behaviors of women and men in committed relationships. But I am doing this deliberately to make a point. Some husbands of women doctors enter marriage with quite a naive and simplistic mind-set; they think that strong, independent, and capable career women do not have emotional needs, that they never feel down or insecure or lonely, and so forth. Consequently, these men do not handle the normal "highs and lows" and emotional vicissitudes of dual career marriages easily, at first. If physician-wives are seriously influenced by their husbands' sanctions against "showing emotion," they will feel harnessed, resentful, and guilty.

In her first visit with me, Dr. Z dropped a lot of hints that made me think she was in conflict about emotional control versus emotional expressiveness. She was very formal and "tight" in her manner toward me. I felt that she expressed more than the usual reserve and tenseness of one's first visit with a psychiatrist. She also made several asides about women and emotions: "My sister's like a yo-yo, very temperamental—her husband calls her hysterical a lot"; "I came home pretty wiped out that day—I saw too many demanding and upset female patients—I guess"; "I suppose you see a lot of women patients yourself as a psychiatrist—don't you find us draining and a pain some days?" As I learned more about Dr. Z's life in this and subsequent visits, I found that her father put her mother down constantly—as well as her and her sister—with one statement: "Your hormones are acting up again." This was not said lightheartedly or humorously, either. Dr. Z described her husband as serious, independent, and self-contained: "He's like a rock—he never has ups and downs. I always feel like a crybaby when I try to discuss personal things with him."

In some marriages of women doctors, this suppression of emotion can, over time, become quite serious. One unhappy woman physician-patient of mine never forgot her husband's words: "I was attracted to your strengths, not your weaknesses." What results is that women in marriages like this develop a code of behavior predicated on being strong and in control at all times. This may become deeply entrenched as a way of being. Women living like this are prone to depression, somatization, and sexual avoidance. When or if they seek psychiatric help, it is essential that their marriages be examined and their husbands interviewed so that appropriate and comprehensive treatment can be given.

WHEN HUSBANDS FEEL BELITTLED

Needless to say, when a husband feels belittled by his physician wife it is extremely important that this feeling be stated and discussed. Its origin may be confusing both for him and his wife. How much of this feeling is his own self-depreciation projected onto her—that is, how much is he putting himself down unconsciously and then blaming her for doing it to him? Does his wife indeed belittle him without being consciously aware of doing so? If she does realize and admit to disparaging him, what are the reasons for her actions? Is she angry at him and attempting to retaliate? Does she feel belittled by him, and are her actions defensive in nature? Has she lost respect for him? Are they so estranged that she no longer cares?

Here are some examples of situations in which husbands of women doctors may feel belittled: when his level of formal education is less than hers (although women in medicine tend to marry men with graduate degrees in the professions, many do not, and these men work in a wide range of occupations); when his work or career is less demanding of time and energy and more easily models a "nine-to-five" job description; when he earns less money than she does; and when his work does not have the same occupational status level as hers. In some of these situations, the husband's feeling of being belittled stems not from within himself or from his wife, but from their extended families, acquaintances, friends, and society at large. The more rigid and conservative their familial and social milieu, the more belittled these husbands may feel.

Several years ago I was referred a young childless couple for marital therapy because of severe communication difficulties, frequent arguments that were becoming physically violent, and sexual disinterest on the husband's part. She was a family physician; he was a letter carrier who had dropped out of college after one semester. Both enjoyed their jobs and clearly respected what the other did for a living. Yet this man frequently felt belittled in the context of their relationship. When this was assessed in more depth, they were able to see that these feelings originated largely from perceived judgments by his family, her family, and many of their friends. Both came from backgrounds where the fathers were more highly educated than the mothers. Their fathers were sole wage earners, and their mothers were home full-time as homemakers and mothers. Also, in their families of origin, both fathers were quite old-fashioned and domineering. Her family felt he might be a "gold digger"; his family teased him for marrying a "rich woman." Their friends, whether in the medical profession or otherwise, taunted them a lot about role reversal, and not always kindly or just in fun.

Some husbands complain that their medical wives employ a double standard with regard to the way that they balance their work and marital commitments. By way of illustration, one man felt that his wife argued that it was fine for her to be late coming home from work, or out several evenings at work-related meetings, or busy on the phone at home because her work involved patients and their medical needs. Yet he felt "attacked" if his work as a landscape artist detained him some evenings or spilled over into their leisure and family time together on evenings and weekends. He argued that his wife did not seem to respect his excuses or rationale for being detained at work as justifiable.

Further discussion of this conflict was very helpful in clarifying their positions and leading to a compromise. She went on to explain that she was trying to protect her personal and marital life (she had been previously divorced) from encroachment by her work by ordering and controlling her medical practice as much as possible. This assertion of control included attempting to have a regular evening meal with a set starting time, plus uninterrupted evenings and weekends whenever possible. As much as her husband lauded her efforts and agreed with them in principle, he still felt controlled, dominated, and treated unfairly. When he explained his need to build up his business in order to bolster his financial and personal security, his wife was able to soften a lot and not be quite as annoyed about his work spilling over into their private time together.

WHEN THE WOMAN PHYSICIAN RESENTS DOING ALL OF THE "WORRY WORK" OF THE MARRIAGE

This complaint is a common one for married women throughout North America. *Worry work* is the term commonly used by women to describe the immense sense of obligation that they feel to monitor and maintain the health of their marriages. Most feel that this responsibility rests squarely on their shoulders and that they receive little or no help from their husbands. As a result, they feel vexed. Women doctors further complain that they have enough on their plates already without having to take on all of this emotional responsibility as well.

More specifically, "worry work" means initiating dialogue about one's marriage from time to time. It means volunteering feelings and statements about one's degree of happiness and unhappiness in marriage. It means asking one's spouse about his or her feelings and level of contentment in the marriage. It includes acknowledging when one is feeling distressed, annoyed, distant, lonely, fearful, and so forth. Suggesting evenings out and weekends away as a couple (plus making the arrangements oneself) is part of the responsibility. Recognizing and acknowledging marital conflict (and lining up a therapist, not just agreeing to come along for the partner's sake) are other examples of "worry work." These are things that many women do single-handedly. They not only become exasperated but also feel sad that their husbands do not seem to care enough to be observant of marital interactions and to seek solutions.

Some women do not mind being the ones to bring up their marriages for discussion, but what annoys them is their husband's lack of responsiveness. Even when his undivided attention is secured, he may have no inkling of what his wife wants to talk about or how to do so. Especially in younger couples this kind of communication may be very difficult and, for the men, quite foreign. The husband may feel he doesn't even know the language, let alone how to be forthcoming with his innermost thoughts and feelings. And yet this is precisely what is requested of him by his wife, for she has either felt quite lonely in her relationship or felt that her husband is not being completely honest with her. For example, most women are able to sense if their husbands are angry with them; yet, in the early stages of many marriages, there are few husbands who are conscious of their anger or, when they are aware of it, are candid enough to admit it to their wives.

In Western society, most husbands do not worry about the "health" of their marriages—witness the number of men each year whose wives leave them. Their wives may leave after years of chaos and unhappiness, but for many of these men, these separations come "out of left field." Witness also the number of men each year who feel dragged or coerced into marital therapy by wives who have threatened to leave them. And witness the number of wives who begin extramarital affairs each year because of marital unhappiness and feelings of being unloved. The men who are most concerned about the health of their marriages are those whose parents divorced, making the men attuned to marital functioning; those who have been married and divorced before and do not want this to happen again; and those who are unusually sensitive to relationship dynamics and whose wives are complacent. Unfortunately, however, rarely do these men directly state to their wives, "I'm unhappy, let's get some counseling"; some say nothing and get depressed, and some start an affair.

Women doctors are more apt to notice and scan articles on marriage in popular magazines, especially those targeted for women readers. Yet most publications written for men do not print articles about marriage; their stories are about sports, business issues, financial planning, computers, and so forth. Occasional articles on divorce highlight the legal and economic aspects only, not the emotional ones. In the medical literature, general medical journals, psychiatric journals, and the *Journal of the American Medical Women's Association* publish papers on the doctor's personal and marital life, but most of the others do not. This is especially so for those specialties whose practitioners are mainly men, such as urology, orthopedic surgery, and neurosurgery. Their journals are restricted to specialty content and do not routinely publish papers about physician health, which is ironic because these are fields that are extremely stressful to one's well-being and marital functioning.

Perhaps much of this is due to a fundamental difference in gender. In this respect Carol Gilligan's research on morality in women and men is instructive. Because, in general, women define morality in terms of relationships and because they take responsibility for themselves and others in relationships, they think and act very differently than men. Men define morality in terms of fairness, in terms of right and wrong. Gilligan's work has a lot of relevance when one stops to consider the seriousness and intensity with which wives and mothers assume their duties and roles in relationship to their husbands and children both through marriage and through divorce.

Let me highlight this issue with an example—one that is quite common in my practice:

Dr. R, a dermatologist, called to ask if I would see her and her husband Dr. E, a radiologist, for "a marriage problem." I made a mental note to myself that she was the one who was placing the call, that is, reaching out and lining up the marital help, even though I had never met her but had met her husband on several occasions (his office was just down the hall from mine). When they came for their first visit, she had a long list of anxious concerns about their relationship. The list made a lot of sense, because their marriage was in serious trouble. They had enormous debts due to some bad investments, they were both drinking too much, they weren't very close anymore and fought a lot, and their

*two youngest children had serious academic and behavioral problems. Un-
like his wife, Dr. E was quite complacent about things: "I'm not so worried about our marriage; I've seen worse. Sharon's always been a worrier—but
I'll come to these sessions if it'll help." His comment made her furious, and she
replied: "How bad do things have to get? Does Carey have to get kicked out of
school again? Do we have to lose our house? Do we have to get cirrhosis of the
liver? And it's not going to help if you just come to these sessions—you have
to work at it!"*

*In our work together, this dynamic came up again and again. Dr. R
complained over and over about how she was fed up carrying all of the
responsibility for the marriage, for her husband's mental and physical health,
and for the children's difficulties. Gradually, Dr. E took on more responsibility
for these things. He arranged meetings with their accountant and tax lawyer,
he set up visits with the children's teachers and counselors, he rearranged his
office hours so they could make appointments with me on Dr. R's day off, and
he became much more attentive and loving at home. This helped tremendously.
Not only did it lighten Dr. R's load, but she began to feel that her husband
cared. She hadn't felt this in a long time. And this shift was good for Dr. E,
too—he was much more involved now in their marriage and family life and less
obsessed with his work.*

WHAT ABOUT THE WOMAN
PHYSICIAN'S CAREER ADVANCEMENT?

The woman physician's career advancement is an extremely important issue that affects marital dynamics in a major way and cuts to the
very heart of a relationship. Examples of opportunities for career advancement include applying for and accepting a residency or competing
for a fellowship in a subspecialty after residency and certification; pursuing an academic tenure-track position over a private opportunity,
thereby foregoing a higher degree of financial remuneration; taking sab-
batical leave or a visiting professorship; presenting papers at national
and international meetings; and serving on time-intensive committees
and holding office on these committees. How do married women doctors and their husbands communicate and come to mutually acceptable
decisions on these matters? How many women doctors never even
consider these sorts of career options because they cannot begin to
imagine their marriages sustaining these pressures and challenges? How
many women doctors suppress and deny their professional dreams and
ambitions because they do not feel (or are not made to feel) that their

career is just as important as their husband's? How many marriages break up over this very basic matter?

We don't have answers to these questions, because we are talking about a relatively new phenomenon (of, say, only the past fifteen years). Never before have there been so many married women doctors in North America. Never before have there been so many opportunities for advanced and highly specialized study. Never before have so many women doctors even considered their rights to a fair hearing in their marriages. As increasing numbers of young couples uproot so that the woman physician can pursue further training, or live in commuter marriages for two to four years, it will be exciting to observe and study the ramifications for husbands and children, as well as illuminating for the medical students and residents who follow.

For many women doctors it boils down to a black-and-white decision: "I had to make a choice; it was either my marriage or my career. I withdrew from the fellowship." What is so crucial for many of these couples is not the actual decision itself but mutuality in coming to the decision. Where there has been good communication, debate, and negotiation in an atmosphere of mature love and trust, both the woman and her husband should feel comfortable with their plans. However, if one or the other feels bullied, threatened, dismissed, or manipulated—and if this is not recognized and aired—then they are in trouble, maybe not immediately, but certainly down the road.

It seems to me that many of the couples who are trying to "do it all," that is, establish and enhance each of their careers plus raise a family, could do with more support and encouragement. I know from my clinical practice that these doctors and their husbands often feel misunderstood and judged by their colleagues, supervisors, friends, and families. A lot of this judgment is rooted in traditional norms about marriage, and some in sexism, but whatever its basis, judgment is not helpful. Navigating in unfamiliar waters, despite the excitement, is always a bit scary.

This was happening for a young couple I saw a couple of years ago for a sexual problem. In the course of their work with me, Alice was accepted to do a two-year fellowship in medical genetics at a major university abroad. She and her husband, Jay, were thrilled. Although he was leaving a very good position with an engineering firm in Vancouver, they had discussed this a lot and were in agreement about Alice's applying for the fellowship. It was the reaction of their family and friends and some of Jay's colleagues at work that surprised them. Jay said, "My father doesn't even understand, and he's a doctor! He feels Alice has enough education already. A couple of guys at work have started to call me 'Mr. Dr. Alice'—I laugh even though it bugs me. And last Saturday night, Alice and I were at a party, and two couples we know came over to us to congratulate Alice. One of the women said, 'You must be quite a guy, Jay—Fred certainly wouldn't give up his job if I wanted to move away to do a fellowship.' I just about died. What do you say in a situation like that?"

WHEN HUSBANDS ARE UNDER- OR UNEMPLOYED

In the 1990s a certain number of women doctors are married to men who cannot find work in their field of study or expertise. Some are unemployed for variable periods of time; others are working at jobs for which they did not train but nevertheless provide some income and some peace of mind. Because these men are working fewer hours per week outside the home as compared to their wives, they generally assume more responsibility for child care and domestic chores. A few are at home full-time, in a role-reversal type of situation in which they care for the children, make the meals, do the shopping, and so forth.

Personal maturity in the woman doctor and her husband and good communication are essential for these marriages to work effectively. Because, in our culture, their respective roles are perceived as deviant, each is subject to outside pressures from colleagues, friends, families, and society at large. And both may have preexisting internal conflict about reversing roles, which is troublesome. Despite today's egalitarian marital norms in the marriages of professional people, they may find themselves thinking and acting in ways that are quite traditional and rooted in their early developmental years.

Barbara and Steve came for marital therapy because of frequent disagreements and arguments, a mutual feeling of "going in different directions," and loss of interest in sex on Barbara's part. Barbara was a family physician, working full-time in a busy, successful, and gratifying private practice. Steve was a classics professor who had been unemployed for three years since being denied tenure at a local university. He was home full-time with their two-and-a-half-year-old son and for the most part enjoyed this. Barbara was six months pregnant. The plan was that she would take one month off after the baby was born, then return to her practice. Steve would continue at home with the two children. Most of the time their arrangement worked extremely well. It was during their fights that Steve expressed his resentment about doing all the work at home and a longing for his own income. Although Barbara had always intended to practice medicine during her child-rearing years, she resented hav-

ing to return to work so quickly after delivery, as well as bearing the entire financial responsibility for the family.

These two did very well with a short course of marital therapy. The key to this therapy was unearthing the way that each felt about what they were doing. Barbara was subject to much criticism from her parents for "marrying a nice but not very practical man," from her women friends for missing her son's "precious years," and even from her patients for "neglecting her son." Steve was made to feel he was a freeloader living off the ambition and finances of his wife. One friend queried the self-respect of a man married to such a "dynamo." And both already felt enough trepidation about how they were leading their lives without the added pressure and judgmental pronouncements of these outside influences.

WHEN THE WOMAN DOCTOR FEELS LIKE AN IMPOSTOR

Transient feelings of being an impostor are not unusual in women doctors, as in other groups of high-achieving women.[20] However, when married women doctors have a deep-seated and pervasive sense of being an impostor, this can become a problem. It is a problem because their husbands simply do not understand. It is rare for men in the professions to have this feeling, and most husbands do not know what their wives are talking about. Most have never heard of the so-called impostor phenomenon (or syndrome) and have not read anything about it.

Women who experience the impostor phenomenon maintain a strong belief that they are not intelligent; in fact, they are convinced that they have fooled anyone who thinks otherwise.[21] Objective evidence of their superior accomplishments does not alter this perception of themselves. These women tend to attribute their success to luck or "fooling the system" as opposed to an inner conviction of ability or talent. At times, this impostor feeling is rooted in personal and family dynamics (e.g., when a young girl receives mixed messages of praise and devaluation from a parent or parents), but not always. Some contemporary women doctors have come of age in a society that associates success and independence with a lack of femininity. Therefore, some women will avoid success so as not to be rejected or have their femininity called into question. More recently, McIntosh has argued for the honesty of people with inner feelings of fraudulence, that perhaps they should be trusted more.[22] She questions the overvalued, "vertical" competitive model of our society as opposed to the undervalued, "horizontal" and collaborative functions in the workplace.

Let me describe a marital conflict around this issue:

Sarah, a twenty-nine-year-old chief resident in internal medicine, was referred on an urgent basis because of severe depression with suicidal thoughts. She responded well to an antidepressant, a two-week leave of absence, and supportive psychotherapy. Once the crisis had passed, she and I were able to uncover the contributing dynamics to her mood change, which included an unresolved problem with her mother and a formal, stiff, and not very intimate marriage. Her husband, Ralph, was a hardworking and dedicated pediatrician who admitted quite openly that he had "trouble with feelings," that he often felt perplexed by Sarah, and apart from medicine felt inadequate compared to her. After some initial anxiety, he quite willingly agreed to marital therapy.

Sarah talked openly about her feelings of being a fake in her residency. These feelings actually dated back to medical school. She believed that her acceptance into medical school was a mistake, that if the admissions committee members truly knew the "real Sarah" they would not have even considered her. She believed that any day soon she'd be called into the department head's office and told, "The jig is up!" Many of her statements were punctuated with references to "fooling them again." Evidence of her academic excellence throughout medical school and residency held little weight in offsetting this feeling of "not cutting it." She countered with, albeit with a wry sense of humor, "If I'm considered one of the better chief residents in this program, heaven help internal medicine in this country."

Sarah had not been able to talk about this impostor feeling with Ralph for years, and she resented him for that. Initially, he attempted to convince her otherwise by logic and the facts of her achievements. He told her repeatedly how clever and competent he felt she was. But because this didn't seem to help, he tried humor and sarcasm. This only made her feel worse and made her more angry. Feeling frustrated and completely shut out, Sarah vowed never to bring it up again. The feelings did not go away; indeed, they worsened. The reassurance and understanding she craved was not forthcoming. When she read an article about the impostor syndrome in a woman's magazine, she decided to show it to Ralph so that he might see that other women have similar sorts of feelings. Ralph's response was dismissive and demeaning; she did not discuss it again until three years later in a conjoint therapy session.

MARRIED WOMEN PHYSICIANS AND DEPRESSION

It has long been known that women are more prone to depression than men. As recently as 1989, large epidemiological and family studies have noted a persistent gender effect, with the risk of depression consistently two to three times higher among women than men across all adult ages.[23]

In the late 1970s, two published psychiatric studies claimed that more than 50% of women physicians suffered from or were at risk for primary affective disorder, that is, clinical depression.[24,25] These studies quite understandably generated considerable response and were found to be severely methodologically flawed, especially in study design and diagnostic criteria constituting a disorder of mood.[26] Further, this research was actually extremely prejudicial against women professionals (i.e., assigning a disease label) and sexist.

I raise the issue in this chapter so that I might argue against reductionism and biomedical skew in assessing women doctors who feel depressed and reach out for professional help. Indeed, as I mentioned earlier, some women physicians will deliberately engage nonmedical therapists over psychiatrists for fear of a diagnostic label and medication. A careful biopsychosocial assessment is absolutely essential—some will be severely depressed with a family history of affective disorder and will need antidepressants and supportive psychotherapy. Some will have underlying intrapsychic conflicts that respond best to insight-oriented, psychodynamic psychotherapy. Some will have interpersonal and marital conflicts; they will need marital or family therapy. Some may need a combination of all of the above, staged and sequenced accordingly.

The combination of depression and marital trouble always requires careful analysis for cause and effect. I will return to this in Chapter Eight on treatment, but I want to register one clinical observation at this point. I am dismayed by the number of depressed women doctors that I have seen in my practice who have been treated previously for depression without their husbands ever being interviewed. These women see themselves as flawed, as do their husbands and previous psychiatrists. Their marriages have not been assessed for possible contributing dynamics; their husbands are not brought into the treatment when they should be. This is especially so when the husbands are doctors, too; they are approached by the psychiatrist as medical colleagues and observers in the field, not as intimately involved marital partners.

Dr. B, an anesthesiologist, and her husband, Dr. F, a pathologist, were referred to me for marital assessment and treatment by Dr. W, a psychiatrist who had been treating Dr. B intermittently for recurrent depression over the previous six years. She had always responded well to antidepressant medicine and to brief supportive psychotherapy. More recently, Dr. B had begun to complain about problems at home, that she and her husband were not communicating very well, that their sexual relationship was less satisfying, and that her husband was drinking more than usual. Dr. W had never met Dr. F before, so he arranged a visit. Dr. F cancelled this visit the day before, saying he was too busy at the hospital. Dr. W did call him and found him "cool and hostile" over the phone. When Dr. W suggested marital treatment, however, Dr. F said he was interested.

What I learned in my first visit with Dr. B and Dr. F was that Dr. F was a very unhappy man. In fact, he was clinically depressed (and suicidal!) himself. I assessed him more thoroughly in an individual visit and started him on an antidepressant. He agreed to stop drinking. It seemed in retrospect that he had actually been depressed for some years, although less severely. He felt that his wife's depressions aggravated his because she was withdrawn and not much fun; she felt that his moods and drinking bouts made her more depressed and hopeless. I told them that I agreed completely with their perceptions and stressed the importance of their both paying attention to their moods and remaining on mood elevators indefinitely. They really didn't need much marital therapy, just reassurance, because I found that they had a viable and functioning marriage most of the time.

WOMEN DOCTORS WHO ARE BATTERED WIVES

The reader's shock and disbelief that a woman doctor could be a battered wife is surpassed only by her shame. Because of this shame, the problem is not easily talked about.[27,28] Therefore, it is difficult to know how common a problem battering is in medical marriages. Some of these women come for treatment on their own when they cannot take it any longer. Although ambivalent, they usually want help in separating from their husbands. Some women have already separated from or divorced their husbands before they are able to talk with anyone about being abused. In fact, I have found that a significant number of women doctors in second marriages describe being battered in their first marriage and give this as their principal reason for leaving the marriage. Some women come with their husbands for marital therapy; the battering may not be revealed at the outset but only later when a trusting, relationship has been established with the therapist. Their husbands' reactions range from complete denial of hitting their wives to an assumption of major responsibility for battering and a commitment to learning ways of changing.

There are many different types of personal and interpersonal dynamics in which violence occurs in marriages of women doctors. The woman may come from an unhappy home in which her father beat her mother and the children. This fact, coupled with a sense of unworthiness and poor self-esteem, may have been influential in her choice of husbands. She may totally lack assertiveness outside the hospital or her practice; she may not even be clear on what is considered acceptable and normative behavior by men in marriages. She may be intimidated by her husband, who indeed may be a physical bully. She gives into his every whim, including sexual whims, to keep the peace and to avoid being struck.

Her husband may be alcoholic; she may find herself making excuses for him, especially if his violent outbursts occur only when he is drinking. As a doctor, she may harbor "rescue fantasies," that is, that she can help him by loving him unconditionally, by giving him what he didn't get in his childhood, and by ensuring he gets good treatment for his alcohol problem. She may have separation anxiety, or fears of loneliness, that win out. In other words, despite marital unhappiness and pain, she opts to stay in her marriage because she feels being with him is better than being alone. She concludes erroneously that she cannot make it on her own. She may have a strong religious conviction to remain in the marriage at all costs, especially when there are children.

Up to this point, I have been talking about battering in the physical sense. What about the woman doctor who is psychologically battered? This can occur in marriages in which the husband is older, more established, and more experienced in relationships. His wife, being younger and having fewer life experiences, is attracted to and awed by his worldliness. It is only after being married a while and maturing herself that the woman begins to question his very convincing and affable authority. She now begins to find him very controlling, but because of the subtle quality of this control, it takes her some time to trust her perceptions. Because he is seen as such a "nice guy" by the world outside, her perceptions are not validated and reinforced by family and friends. They do not understand what she is complaining about; she begins to feel guilty and wonders if she is going crazy. Meanwhile, she continues to feel herself slowly dying inside, becoming withdrawn and depressed.

In a similar way, this type of woman also becomes a victim of marital rape. She has never had an understanding of or appreciation for her own, personally constructed sexual needs. If she does come to some realization of her likes and dislikes, her attempts to communicate them to her husband lack assertiveness and strength. And given his personality, he does not listen or overrules her anyway. Defeated, she continues to just give in and to accommodate him sexually; she derives no pleasure, or fakes pleasure, and the charade is upheld. Eventually she becomes numb.

This portrait of the emotionally battered woman doctor is not rare. Many of these women do not come to understand their situation until their marriage is on its last legs. Some see the dynamics only after divorce and in retrospect as they reflect on the marital issues several years later. Many come to these insights only through their evolving personal feminism, and it may not be until this time that they are able to talk about it. Their connection and engagement with other women whom they respect and believe in enable them to transcend the embarrassment and shame.

WOMEN DOCTORS WITH PREGNANCY COMPLICATIONS

Pregnancy can be a stressful time for any couple, especially if there are medical difficulties. Women physicians may have trouble conceiving and then have pregnancy complications because of delayed childbearing associated with such a long course of study and training. In a study of thirty-seven physicians, Schwartz found that her patients were about five years older than average at the time of pregnancy and that most of them continued to work until they went into labor.[29] Further, she noted an increased incidence of preterm labor, a higher incidence of abruptio placentae, and hence an increased rate of cesarean section.

Pregnant women physicians may develop marital symptoms if their pregnancy is high risk. Not only is fear of losing the pregnancy a stressor in itself, but this anxiety may upset a couple's marital equilibrium. More specifically, having to stop work earlier than expected may mean loss of income, an interruption in one's training, worries about coverage of one's patients, increased work load for medical colleagues, and social isolation. The ability of the woman's husband to adapt and cope with added responsibilities is an important factor. Even the happiest of married couples can feel very tense, demoralized, less intimate, and irritable living with a complicated pregnancy.

Here is an example:

Dr. B, a forty-year-old pediatrician, called me from her room at a local maternity hospital where she had been admitted. She had come into the hospital two weeks earlier because of premature labor and leaking amniotic fluid; hence, she was on complete bed rest until she went into labor or it could be safely induced. She said she was in the midst of a marital crisis. When I visited her, I learned that her husband had left the day before to go to Club Med "to find himself." Needless to say, Dr. B felt very frightened, abandoned, and furious.

Her husband called her the next day from Mexico, full of embarrassment and remorse, and with a change of plans to fly home that evening. I spoke to him the following day. He was quite an immature man who had a history of impulsive behavior. He felt terrible about what he had done and agreed with his wife that they did have a very solid marriage.

I had a few visits with the two of them together after their baby was born just to make certain they were adjusting satisfactorily, which they were. Looking back, both of them identified many worries that they had been sitting on throughout the pregnancy and had not been discussing. Most especially, she was concerned about balancing her busy schedule as a solo pediatrician in their community once the baby arrived. And he was worried about finances, given that his business was not doing well and he might have to declare bankruptcy.

MARRIED WOMEN PHYSICIANS AND SUBSTANCE ABUSE

I mentioned in Chapter Two that alcohol abuse and self-medicating in male physicians are more often the cause of marital difficulty than the result. This applies to women physicians as well, although I occasionally see couples wherein the woman physician's drinking or drug-taking is clearly secondary to an acute marital mishap of some sort; once the crisis is past, the behavior stops.

In an interview study of ninety-five women physicians and five women medical students who were self-described alcoholics, Bissell and Skorina noted some important findings.[30] Only 40% were addicted to alcohol alone, and most had felt suicidal prior to sobriety (about one third had made suicide attempts). The presence of alcoholism in the nuclear family and marital instability were common. What is striking is how few of these women were diagnosed and referred for treatment by their personal physicians or therapists or by their state impaired-physician committees. The reason for the latter finding may be the fact that many physician support committees do not have women physician representation, and the authors suggest that this imbalance be addressed. More emphatically, Steindler urges the leaders in organized medicine to reach out to women physicians with acts of collegial regard and compassion "to make the house of medicine their home."[31]

Now that clinicians have a greater understanding of dual diagnosis (i.e., substance abuse coexisting with psychiatric illnesses such as depression, panic disorder, and obsessive–compulsive disorder), women physicians who drink excessively or take sedatives and painkillers should receive more comprehensive assessment and treatment. This should include a fair assessment of their marriages and marital therapy if indicated because, not unlike wives of chemically dependent physicians, husbands and children of alcoholic women physicians often feel very confused and powerless.

Dr. J and her husband, Dr. T, came for marital therapy at her request. He was reluctant to come, saying to her, "Now that you're not drinking, aren't we happy?" Dr. J was very lonely in her marriage and felt that her husband's first two loves were medicine (he was a family physician) and sailing. She saw herself and the children as third on her husband's priorities.

Dr. J, a psychiatrist, had been drinking heavily for at least ten years before she sought treatment. In fact, it was a classmate of hers who was instrumental in getting the local physician support committee to do an intervention. Her husband didn't think her drinking was "that bad." This was largely because he was never around. Dr. J entered detoxification and residential treatment, followed by weekly attendance at a physicians' support group. She also attended AA and IDAA.

When the two of them came for marital therapy, Dr. J had been sober for three years. Her husband was quite psychologically unsophisticated and really had no insight into what it takes to be an involved husband and father. Working with him was a challenge. He was sincere, albeit a bit slow, in his efforts to change his life-style and to be less self-centered. After about a dozen marital therapy visits, he was beginning to become more organized in his office and to get home for dinner. He also took more interest in his children's schoolwork and activities. He spontaneously remembered Dr. J's birthday and planned an evening out, which meant a lot to her. It also meant a lot to Dr. T when his wife, without any prompting from him, signed up for sailing lessons.

CONCLUSION

I have outlined here some of the more common complaints and findings in troubled marriages of women doctors. One can see that these concerns exist on many different levels—those on the surface are more straightforward; others, at a deeper level, are more complex. There are biological, psychological, and sociocultural factors that give these marriages their unique and particular design, but I have not been able to discuss all of these determinants. These case studies are just a beginning. As more and more women study and practice medicine, we will have a better understanding of the complexity and diversity of their marriages.

REFERENCES

1. Judith Lorber, "Sisterhood Is Synergistic," *Journal of the American Medical Women's Association* 41 (July/August 1986), 116–119.
2. Malkah T. Notman and Carol C. Nadelson, "Medicine: A Career Conflict for Women," *American Journal of Psychiatry* 130 (October 1973), 1123–1126.

3. Merville O. Vincent, M. Margaret Hill, and M. Ruth Tatham, "The Physician's Marriage, Husband, Family and Practice," *Ontario Medical Review* (July 1976), 350–356.

4. Marcia Angell, "Women in Medicine: Beyond Prejudice," *New England Journal of Medicine* 304 (May 7, 1981), 1161–1163.

5. Leon Eisenberg, "The Distaff of Aesculapius—The Married Woman as Physician," *Journal of the American Medical Women's Association* 36 (February 1981), 84–88.

6. Carola Eisenberg, "Women as Physicians," *Journal of Medical Education* 58 (July 1983), 534–541.

7. Judith Lorber, *Women Physicians: Career, Status, and Power* (New York: Tavistock, 1984).

8. Carol C. Nadelson and Malkah T. Notman, "The Woman Physician's Marriage," in *Medical Marriages*, ed. Glen O. Gabbard and Roy W. Menninger (Washington, D.C.: American Psychiatric Press, 1988), 79–88.

9. Bonnie J. Tesch, Janet Osborne, Deborah E. Simpson, Sara F. Murray, and Joanna Spiro, "Women Physicians in Dual-Physician Relationships Compared with Those in Other Dual-Career Relationships," *Academic Medicine* 67 (August 1992), 542–544.

10. Wendy Levinson, Susan W. Tolle, and Charles Lewis, "Women in Academic Medicine: Combining Career and Family," *New England Journal of Medicine* 321 (November 30, 1989), 1511–1517.

11. P. Uhlenberg and T. M. Cooney, "Male and Female Physicians: Family and Career Comparisons," *Social Science in Medicine* 30 (March 1990), 373–378.

12. Michael F. Myers, "Overview. The Female Physician and Her Marriage," *American Journal of Psychiatry* 141 (November 1984), 1386–1391.

13. Michael F. Myers, "Doctors' Spouses and Doctors as Spouses," *Canadian Family Physician* 32 (February 1986), 327–329.

14. Michael F. Myers, "Marital Issues for Women Physicians," *Annals of the Royal College of Physicians and Surgeons of Canada* 19 (March 1986), 101–104.

15. Michael F. Myers, *Men and Divorce* (New York: Guilford, 1989), 50–51.

16. Michael F. Myers, "Treating Physicians with Psychotherapy," *Directions in Psychiatry* 12 (June 26, 1992), 1–8.

17. Carol Gilligan, *In a Different Voice: Psychological Theory and Women's Development* (Cambridge, Mass.: Harvard University Press, 1982).

18. Gordon Parker and Roslyn Jones, "The Doctor's Husband," *British Journal of Medical Psychology* 54 (1981), 143–147.

19. Michael F. Myers, "Overview: The Female Physician and Her Marriage," *American Journal of Psychiatry* 141 (November 1984), 1386–1391.

20. Pauline R. Clance and Suzanne A. Imes, "The Impostor Phenomenon in High Achieving Women: Dynamics and Therapeutic Intervention," *Psychotherapy: Theory, Research and Practice* 15 (Fall 1978), 241–247.

21. David W. Krueger, *Success and the Fear of Success in Women* (New York: Free Press, 1984), 86–91.

22. Peggy McIntosh, *Feeling Like a Fraud* (Work in Progress Series, Stone Center for Developmental Services and Studies, Wellesley, Mass.: Wellesley College, 1985).

23. Gerald L. Klerman and Myrna M. Weissman, "Increasing Rates of Depression," *Journal of the American Medical Association* 261 (April 21, 1989), 2229–2235.

24. Amos Welner, Sue Marten, Eliza Wochnik, Mary A. Davis, Roberta Fishman, and Paula J. Clayton, "Psychiatric Disorders Among Professional Women," *Archives of General Psychiatry* 36 (February 1979), 169–173.

25. Ferris N. Pitts, Jr., Arthur B. Schuller, Charles L. Rich, and Andrew F. Pitts, "Suicide Among U.S. Women Physicians, 1967–1972," *American Journal of Psychiatry* 136 (May 1979), 694–696.

26. Gabrielle A. Carlson and Diana C. Miller, "Suicide, Affective Disorder, and Women Physicians," *American Journal of Psychiatry* 138 (October 1981), 1330–1335.
27. Janet A. Whitehall, "Wife," *Journal of the American Medical Association* 261 (June 16, 1989), 3460.
28. G. L. Bundow, "Why Women Stay," *Journal of the American Medical Association* 267 (June 17, 1992), 3229.
29. Ruth W. Schwartz, "Pregnancy in Physicians: Characteristics and Complications," *Obstetrics and Gynecology* 66 (November 1985), 672–676.
30. LeClair Bissell and Jane Skorina, "One Hundred Alcoholic Women in Medicine: An Interview Study," *Journal of the American Medical Association* 257 (June 5, 1987), 2939–2944.
31. Emanuel M. Steindler, "Alcoholic Women in Medicine: Still Homeless," *Journal of the American Medical Association* 257 (June 5, 1987), 2954–2955.

Chapter Four

GAY AND LESBIAN
PHYSICIAN COUPLES

The percentage of medical students and physicians who are gay and lesbian remains largely unknown, because open acknowledgment of homosexuality is a step taken by very few members of the medical profession. Nevertheless, whatever the numbers, many gay men and lesbian women in medicine form and maintain long-standing relationships with their partners. They too are subject to particular stresses, both from within and without. In this chapter, I will outline some of their concerns.

Like their married heterosexual colleagues, gay and lesbian medical students and physicians share certain generic problems in their relationships. They may have difficulty communicating with each other, which leads to tension, frustration, and unhappiness. There may be frequent arguments and fighting, including physical violence. They may have conflicts with their own and each other's families, especially around matters of acceptance of their relationship. There may be money worries. Alcoholism and abuse of other drugs may complicate and jeopardize their commitment to each other. They may develop a sexual problem, and any one of the various dysfunctions is possible. Finally, there may be a crisis precipitated by infidelity—which classically is more common in gay males than lesbian couples. Since the advent of AIDS (Acquired Immune Deficiency Syndrome), most gay male couples are monandrous.

Although the complaints and problems of gay male and lesbian couples are similar to those of married heterosexuals, there are significant differences in the *form* the relationships take. Gay and lesbian relationships are more commonly structured along egalitarian lines. Both partners are considered equal in many if not most ways. In traditional marriages there is a power differential; the man, as breadwinner, holds the power. In dual career marriages, there is less of a power differential, but it still exists, even with women enjoying the same status and income as their husbands. When there is a power disparity in gay male or lesbian couples it is not based on gender but on other differences such as age, education, occupation, or financial position.

Another major difference in the form of gay and lesbian relationships is that they are not legally sanctioned. There is no marriage license. There is no actual marriage ceremony or wedding. The union is not celebrated, except in rare instances when the two individuals exchange vows and rings in the presence of close friends (a commitment ceremony). There is no legal authorization, although there are now statutes to protect each individual's assets and property rights in case of separation.

Although the American Civil Liberties Union has issued a formal policy statement seeking elimination of legal barriers to homosexual marriages,[1] and others have spoken out in support of gay marriage,[2,3] there is a powerful backlash against the social acceptance of homosexuality.[4,5] The psychological significance of this basic attitudinal difference toward gay and lesbian couples (versus heterosexual couples) must not be underestimated.

SOCIAL PREJUDICE

There is tremendous social disapproval of homosexual people in North America, and this has increased markedly since the 1980s. Two major reasons for this are the movement toward moral and religious conservatism and society's reaction to the frightening disease AIDS. Overt prejudice such as the return of the sodomy laws in some states and an outcry against civil rights bills to prohibit discrimination in employment, housing, and public accommodations on the basis of sexual orientation is only the manifest evidence of this increasing homophobia (i.e., irrational fear of homosexuality). This is a serious step backward for the gay-affirmative movement of the 1960s and 1970s, which included the beginning of gay and lesbian acceptance in North America.

But does this national or global change directly affect the specific couple? Can't they "insulate" themselves against people who do not accept their lifestyle? Can't they move to their own community or enclave (translate "ghetto")? Why don't they turn the other cheek? These are all examples of questions based in ignorance and fear. The fact of the matter is that all minority groups are intensely affected by these kinds of attitudes.

The following provides a very simple but vivid example of the pernicious effects of gay-bashing:

A few years ago I was treating a gay medical student, Sam, and his partner of three years, Tom. Their main problem was a sexual one that was rooted in Sam's having been severely sexually assaulted some years earlier while an adolescent. In one session they arrived feeling furious, dejected, and not speaking to each other. They gave an account of a major argument they had had forty-eight hours earlier that included a lot of name-calling, mudslinging, "hitting below the belt," and so forth. I was taken aback by all of this because they had been doing very well for several weeks. When I asked about possible precipitants, initially they could not think of anything; they had been out walking the entire day and enjoying each other's company. Then Tom mentioned an incident that occurred as they were nearing their home. A carload of young men pulled up to the curb and started taunting them with suggestive antigay remarks and gestures. One yelled out, "Hi girls, want some real *men?" They didn't persist and quickly drove off, as Sam and Tom tried to ignore them and dismiss the entire experience. But they weren't able to forget. The statements of the men in the car upset their equilibrium and provoked their own internal homophobia with resultant upset and retaliatory rage, which they took out on each other. Both ended up feeling emotionally bruised and battered and completely demoralized about their future together.*

Social sanction and support are fundamental to the growth and stability of coupled people. Almost always do married couples have the acceptance and blessing of their families, friends, acquaintances at work, and even neighbors. Many also have religion and its pastorate as a resource in times of marital and family upset. By way of contrast, most gay male and lesbian couples do not have this sustenance. Their families often do not accept their relationship, at least at first, or perhaps a sibling does but the parents do not. Even when they come around to accepting, some parents feel very awkward in demonstrating their love and care, or give mixed messages, for example, inviting their daughter's partner to a small family dinner but not to their son's wedding.

In some communities with very few gay or lesbian people, the couple may feel intensely lonely and isolated. If they are quite closeted about their homosexuality that makes it even more difficult, because there will be no close couple friends—whether gay, lesbian, or straight—for support, companionship, leisure, and venting of normal and every-day problems.

Without this measure of acceptance from others, the couple itself becomes the refuge, the retreat from the world. An attitude of "it's us against them" develops as a self-protective and defensive stance. This may work at first, especially in the early months of a relationship, when the two individuals are cementing attachment bonds anyway. But this becomes insular over time. Too many needs have to be met, or are expected to be met, by each other. This insularity leads to tension and frustration, feelings of disappointment, and feelings of suffocation. Further, there is a betrayed and lonely feeling if one's partner reaches out to others. Irritated and hostile, the two individuals begin to sense they are destroying each other.

Like childless married couples, gay male and lesbian couples do not have children as a common central point, a shared purpose, a generative extension of themselves. This can contribute to this feeling and expectation of having to be "all things to each other." Those people who are well integrated socially, both as individuals and as a couple, and who tend to be fairly open with others, will not experience this problem. One lesbian woman who was considering artificial insemination said, "I really am torn about having a child. In addition to my intense desire to be a mother, I feel strongly that a son or daughter would help Clara and me to focus our love, to become more engaged, and to unite together. However, when we're not getting along, and I want to leave, I realize how much simpler and less painful it is to separate without children."

I want to talk now about relationship concerns and problems that are unique to gay male couples and those that are unique to lesbian couples. This raises several questions about the formation, evolution, and maintenance of a love relationship between two people of the same sex. Unlike men and women who meet and come together with vastly different biological and psychosocial experiences, based on gender alone, that date back to birth, we are now considering two men or two women meeting, falling in love, and forming a commitment to each other. In what ways are they complementary and in what ways similar? And what is the distribution and balance of complementarity and similarity in their relationship? How does this translate into how they court, communicate, express emotion, show affection, make love, share domestic chores, manage their finances, and so forth? In what ways are their values, expectations, and behavioral norms similar to and different from married couples?

GAY MALE COUPLES

COMPETITION

According to sex-role socialization theory, men are socialized from boyhood to be independent, autonomous, strong, and competitive, that is, instrumental.[6] Therefore, men in a love relationship with each other, because they are of the same gender, will have these traits and strivings coloring their interactions and behavior together. The positive aspects of this are enhancing; each may be stimulated toward personal fulfillment and accomplishment. As a couple, they are seen as exciting and dynamic individuals.

However, these same characteristics can cause problems. In my clinical work with gay male couples, I have found competition with each other a common complaint as a destructive element. I think it is both a cause of problems (i.e., inherent male competition leads to feeling unsupported and distant) and a result of problems (i.e., being beset with problems and feeling misunderstood brings out a competitive need to regain one's self-pride and self-esteem). Arenas of competition include the usual "male" ones—money, intelligence, success in the job market, sports, sexual prowess—and others as well. Partners may compete over their looks, their physiques, their attractiveness to other men, their platonic male friends, their culinary skills, or their taste in art and design, to name a few areas. As one can see, these are all surface issues—underlying these, each man may have fears of commitment, separation, or isolation as well as problems with intimacy and self-esteem.

Before AIDS, many gay male couples were open to sexual expression outside the core union.[7] This was considered a norm and a standard that set gay male couples apart from lesbian couples (wherein non-monogamy is rare) and certainly from heterosexual couples (except for the brief popularity of "open marriage" during the 1970s). But even then, many gay men in couples were unhappy and threatened by outside sex. For them, these sexual liaisons were indicative of a problem at home, did not enhance the primary relationship, and in fact were destructive and caused more problems.

SEXUAL ACTING OUT

As in heterosexual couples, sexual "acting out" often means a breakdown in verbal communication. I have seen this repeatedly in gay male couples. Men in general are not readily in touch with their feelings, that is, the feelings appropriate to an event or thought are not as easily accessible. When men experience feelings, their ability to openly express them does not come easily. Historically, men have not been socialized while growing up to talk about their feelings, especially "softer" and tender ones. In general, women are more adept than men at anticipating feelings in others and inviting them to disclose these feelings openly. Usually, they listen better. With this as background, it is easier to understand why and how verbal communication between men who love each other frequently goes awry.

Paul and Ben came for therapy because of extreme tension at home, constant bickering, and mutual bewilderment as to why this was happening. Both wanted to separate unless something changed. Paul was a senior resident in dermatology; Ben was a pharmacist. They had known each other for four years and had been living together for three years. In the initial visit, in which I saw them together, I learned that Ben had had a brief "fling" with another man one year earlier. This was the first and only time that either had been sexually active outside their relationship, which they defined as "open with discretion." Neither felt that Ben's involvement with this other man had any relevance to their present difficulties.

I suggested individual sessions with each of them. These visits were illuminating. In addition to discussing their personal and family backgrounds, both focused on Ben's outside sexual liaison. Ben admitted to feeling increasingly inferior to Paul as the latter progressed through residency. He found Paul becoming increasingly confident and knowledgeable, which he liked, but also a bit arrogant. He also found him increasingly self-absorbed with work and study—he wasn't as much fun anymore and was becoming "too serious." Ben did not like and feel comfortable with many of Paul's friends and associates from work. Despite Paul's attempts at reassurance, Ben did not feel accepted by these people. His efforts to discuss these matters with Paul were met with defensiveness and statements that he was being "hypersensitive." Ben began to go out more on his own, especially when Paul was on call, and one night at a bar met the man with whom he became involved. After seeing him twice, Ben became so alarmed at the intensity of his feelings that he stopped calling his new acquaintance.

In his individual visit, Paul admitted to unresolved feelings about Ben's affair. He had bothersome recurrent images of Ben and this other man in bed together. He had asked Ben for specific details of what they actually did in bed, but Ben refused to tell him. Paul was not only surprised at his reaction to Ben's being with someone else but expected the feelings to pass quickly. He was troubled that he felt hurt, anger, and jealousy at all, let alone that he still felt these emotions one year later. He had not discussed any of this with Ben.

What this clinical example illustrates is the difficulty that these two men had in communicating soft and vulnerable feelings to one another. At different times in their relationship, they each felt shut out, hurt, and resentful. Both tried to remain cool and in control at the expense of their true feelings. Both backed away quickly when they didn't feel heard and felt misunderstood. Both wanted to avoid open confrontation and to preserve their calm equilibrium.

FEARS OF INTIMACY

Gay men in relationships may have difficulties with intimacy that may range all the way from talking about personal feelings to making a commitment to the relationship. Depending on the intensity of their need for autonomy, they may associate intimacy with weakness or dependence. They may not realize that it is quite possible, if not desirable, to have a good measure of both autonomy and intimacy in a healthy and stable relationship.

Prohibitions against intimacy and fears of intimacy, when they exist in a gay male couple, are always manifest in their sexual relationship. This sounds like a paradox at first, because sex is generally considered such an intimate act; yet sex can actually be a defense against intimacy. Sex can be used to avoid or short-circuit verbal communication, self-disclosure, and problem solving. Complaints such as the following are revealing: "We fuck constantly, but we don't make love anymore"; "There's no foreplay, we just get it on"; "I don't come as easily anymore, sometimes not at all"; "Since I played around on him last year, I swear he's rougher in bed with me"; "I haven't felt like sex in years—I just let him do me."

Men in situations like these can benefit a lot from therapy. The dynamics of their sexual life together can be analyzed, and blocked feelings can be validated and expressed. Further, the therapist can assist them in putting into words what they are feeling, or not feeling, when they are being sexual together. The goal is enjoyable and intimate sexual communication, not mechanical and performance-oriented sex devoid of feelings. Their verbal communication will also improve in depth and effectiveness.

"COMING OUT" PROBLEMS

Coming out refers to the process of acquiring and accepting a homosexual identity.[8] It begins with self-acceptance and then includes disclosure to others, who may be close friends, family, people at work, and sometimes society at large, that is, "going public." Men who are gay vary tremendously along this axis of self-acceptance and self-disclosure, and men in couples do as well. This can present a problem and lead to friction in the relationship.

Tim and Frank, physicians in their thirties, had been together for six years. Tim had been married before, and he defined himself as having come out toward the end of his marriage when he met Frank. He disclosed his homosexuality to

his wife, and after several months of pain and unhappiness for both of them,
they separated and divorced. By this time, Tim had told his parents, siblings,
and many friends and work associates about his homosexuality.

Frank, on the other hand, was very closeted. He had never discussed his
homosexuality with his parents, who lived in another city. He had no brothers
or sisters. He was very private in his personal and social life and preferred to
keep this totally separate from his work life. In fact, to ensure this he deliber-
ately accepted a salaried position in an adjacent community, to which he
commuted daily. Before he met Tim, he was friendly with only three people, a
gay man and a lesbian couple; the four of them formed a tight group and did
many things socially.

One of the reasons Tim and Frank began to fight with each other was
because they had become polarized on the coming-out issue. Neither could
understand the other's position; each felt hurt, controlled, and stonewalled by
the other. When Frank's parents came to stay with them, Tim hated playing the
charade that they were roommates with separate bedrooms. When Tim's parents
visited, Frank felt that Tim deliberately tried to "embarrass" him by calling him
"sweetheart" or attempting to hold his hand in their presence. Although he
knew that Tim's parents accepted and loved the two of them, Frank continued
to feel self-conscious and formal when they were around.

There is another aspect of coming out that can cause distress in a
gay male couple. If one partner is in the very early stages of this
process, which can take years, he may find himself taking three steps
forward and two steps backward for a long time. He comes to doubt
whether he really is gay or whether this is what he wants (as if he has
full control over it) or wonders if he might actually be bisexual or a
late-blooming heterosexual. He may have mood swings. For many periods of time he is happy, secure, and confident about his sexuality; other
times he is depressed, guilty, and full of self-doubts. If his partner has
been comfortably gay for years, or perhaps did not have as much difficulty coming out, he will experience a lot of emotional upset in the
relationship. Indeed, his patience and sympathy will wear thin; he may
become frustrated, resentful, sarcastic, or despondent. Underneath, he
may also fear abandonment.

AGE DISCREPANCY

There may be a significant difference in age between the two men
in some gay relationships, a difference spanning ten to fifteen years at
times. This may or may not be a problem. I wonder sometimes if these
relationships are more troublesome for the friends and families of these

couples than for the two individuals themselves. In the first place, cynicism about the viability and continuance of gay men in couples abounds in our society, both inside and outside of the gay community. And second, when one man is quite a bit older than the other, stereotypic thinking imagines that they are playing father-son roles, that the younger is being "kept" by the older.

The dynamics of such a couple are not unlike those of a heterosexual couple in which there is an older man and younger woman. In essence, the younger partner is attracted to and respects the emotional and occupational stability of the older man. He may see him as a bit of a role model and as a man with life experiences and wisdom. He probably feels safe and secure with him, something he may not have felt in earlier relationships with men his own age. The older partner is attracted to the younger man's promise and potential. He enjoys his youthfulness and playfulness, which he may feel keeps him young and in touch. He finds him physically appealing and sexually exciting. Both discount their chronological age difference—the younger sees the older as "not your typical forty-year-old" and the older sees the younger as "a very mature twenty-five-year-old."

Robert was a forty-two-year-old pathologist who presented for treatment with a serious clinical depression. He responded well to tricyclic antidepressants and supportive psychotherapy. Once he was asymptomatic, we began insight-oriented therapy in which he worked through long-standing problems with his father, older brother, internalized homophobia, and unresolved grief from a five-year relationship that had ended one year before consulting me. Toward the end of his therapy with me, he met a twenty-three-year-old university student, Matthew. Their relationship moved along very quickly, and after three months Matthew moved into Robert's home.

Approximately six months after my work with Robert ended, he called requesting to see me again. His main complaint was a return of depressive feelings, broken sleep, panicky feelings in the night and early morning, and loss of interest in sex. He denied problems in the relationship, but he feared that Matthew would leave him if he didn't "straighten up." I diagnosed a recurrent depression, which responded to a few psychotherapy visits. Medication was not necessary. An individual visit with Matthew confirmed the change in Robert's mood; I found him to be sensitive and supportive. He was very committed to the relationship and had no thoughts of leaving Robert. He also felt that much of Robert's "insecurity" was because most of their friends and associates joked about the two of them, made value judgments, and couldn't see them lasting as a couple more than a year.

However, there can be conflicts in couples with a significant age difference. One central dynamic may be related to power and control, similar to what adolescent sons experience with their fathers. Given that each individual is at a different life stage, the younger man may want and need more freedom and independence in the relationship, and the older man may be threatened by this. Or the older man may expect or demand a level of maturity and structure in his partner that the latter cannot and will not meet. Like an adolescent, the younger man may also act out against perceived "parental" control and limit setting by staying out late, not communicating, drinking, not saving money, and so forth. Consequently, both end up feeling hurt, disappointed, and resentful.

GAY FATHERS

Men in gay relationships may have been married before and one partner, occasionally both, may have children from that marriage.[9] Most often these men are noncustodial fathers, but there are situations in which a gay father has custody and has the children living with him (and his partner, if he is in a cohabiting relationship). Let me discuss the former situation, because it is more common.

As in all stepfamily situations, the roles are ambiguous and confusing for all parties, especially at the beginning. The children, depending on their ages, may or may not have been told of their dad's sexual orientation. Consequently, they may or may not know the nature of their dad's relationship with his friend and "roommate." Most gay fathers in relationships want to include their partners in activities when they see their children, some or perhaps most of the time. Many ex-wives of gay men are still hurting and are bitter in the early months or years after separation. They do not want their children exposed to "the homosexual life-style" and they may forbid access unless their former husbands comply. This in turn infuriates these fathers, who may have no recourse but to accommodate their ex-wives' wishes or to fight it out in court. This adds fuel to the fire of the already tenuous coparenting relationship between the children's mother and father.

The impact of all of this on the gay couple is enormous. First of all, they do not feel accepted as a mature and loving couple who can provide responsible and proper care to the children. They are seen as deviant, incapable, or harmful. With restrictions on access to their children, these men do not feel they are allowed to be complete fathers, or honest fathers. The frustration and anger that is generated over all of this may spill over into the relationship with their life partner, causing tension, misunderstanding, and fighting at home. For some men there is residual self-loathing just below the surface about being gay; it can be easily reactivated with this type of pressure.

Second, some children will not want to know the true nature of their dad's relationship with his friend. They are happy enough to know that Dad has a close friend, and most of the time they will enjoy doing things with him as well. Adolescent children who know their father is gay will have a tightly guarded secret that they share with only their closest and most trusted of friends. They may go through alternating periods of accepting and rejecting their father and his partner. Open and persistent attempts at communication are crucial during this period.

Finally, there may be friction if the gay father's partner cannot come to terms with sharing the man he loves. In other words, he sees the children as an intrusion, and he feels that they take something from him, as opposed to enhancing his life. He may be jealous of the time his partner spends with his children, and he will feel shortchanged. Of course, the gay father feels torn and caught in the middle: he loves his children, and he loves his partner. Unless a compromise can be reached, they may need to separate. This type of issue is very similar to what occurs in heterosexual remarried couples when the time (both quantitative and qualitative) that the man spends with his children from an earlier marriage is upsetting to his wife.

AIDS

Within the gay community, the specter of AIDS is being experienced with an immediacy that is not yet present in many sectors of the heterosexual community.[10] Most gay men who live in cities where AIDS is prevalent, such as New York and San Francisco, have lost several friends and acquaintances to AIDS. Many have lost life partners or will.

What are some of the issues for gay couples when one or both have AIDS? Loss is ever present. There is loss of health and physical livelihood as the disease progresses. There is loss of economic security when one has to quit work and at the same time cope with medical expenses. There may be loss of sexuality and perhaps intimacy within the relationship; in fact, the relationship itself might end because of so much stress in both partners. There is loss of privacy as one's sexual orientation and illness become known to family members, friends, employers, workmates, hospital personnel, and often neighbors. There is loss of one's confidence and self-esteem living with the stigma attached to AIDS. There is loss of one's autonomy, and sometimes one's dignity, while fighting dependency on others for care, comfort, and nurturance. And there may be loss of one's loved ones (i.e., friends or a life partner) to AIDS while trying to fight death oneself.

It may be very difficult to talk about these matters because they are so painful and so sad. Here is an example of blocked communication:

Ed and William, a couple in their mid-thirties, had already separated when they came to see me. Ed was a family physician who had stopped working six months earlier because of extreme weight loss and exhaustion associated with AIDS. William was a college professor who also had HIV, but he was well and working full-time. They had been together for two years, having met in a support group for HIV-infected people. They both had the same complaint: "We can't talk to each other anymore."

What I learned in my first visit with them and in visits that I had with each of them alone was that both of them were sitting on many feelings that they were afraid or unable to discuss. Ed felt completely shut out when he tried to talk about anything to do with death or dying, such as his will, his rapid worsening and weakness, his failing vision (due to cytomegalic viral retinitis), his loss of interest in sex (and his guilt about this), and his worry about William's health after his death. William had a lot of feelings and fears about losing Ed and angrily felt that the latter was giving in and giving up. He also felt guilty that he couldn't do more to help—to take Ed to doctor's appointments, to cook better meals, and to make him laugh more. He worried while he was at work that Ed might fall or miss meals or perhaps even commit suicide.

Couple therapy was extremely helpful in facilitating what needed to be discussed. They regained their closeness very quickly and immediately resumed living together, to the relief of each. And they remained together in a very loving and mutually respectful way until Ed's death nine months later.

LESBIAN COUPLES

CONFLICTS OF CLOSENESS AND DISTANCE

Conflicts of closeness and distance are very common in lesbian couples who present for treatment. This is well documented in the published literature.[11] *Fusion* is the term used to describe the sense of embeddedness and loss of the individual self that is felt, and feared, by lesbian women in close monogamous relationships. Its polar opposite, complete separateness and distance, is equally frightening and unacceptable. Finding a middle ground, with a comfortable balance of togetherness and individual autonomy, is particularly difficult for many lesbian couples.

This "tightness" of couples is commonly a reaction to the lack of acceptance by the heterosexual world; they erect and maintain rigid boundaries in order to preserve their integrity and validity as a couple. This behavior is the "it's us against them" stance I described earlier in this chapter. Intense and defensive bonding is much less prominent in lesbian couples who are accepted by their respective families and who are well integrated in the lesbian and heterosexual communities.

Also helpful in understanding women in lesbian relationships is the gender-specific research of the past fifteen years, commonly called "the new psychology of women." Miller has described the tendency of women to inhibit and suppress their aggressive and competitive desires because of their fear of hurting others and isolating themselves.[12] Gilligan's work on morality finds women defining themselves in terms of relationships and taking responsibility and care in relationships with others.[13] With these observations and findings in mind, it is easier to appreciate the difficulties that two women in a love relationship might have in clearly communicating their needs and wishes to each other.

Unfortunately, not all therapists have incorporated these ideas, with their interpersonal, feminist, and systems theory underpinnings, into their work with women in lesbian relationships. They use value-laden terms and concepts—*overly dependent, neurotic, masochistic, clinging, symbiotic,* and so forth—in their dynamic understanding and treatment approaches.

These values were vividly illustrated in my initial visit with a twenty-eight-year-old medical student whose chief complaint was, "I guess I just like to suffer." When I asked her what she meant by that, she went on to describe a complicated and unhappy relationship with another woman who was severely alcoholic. They had been together for five years. Two years earlier she had consulted another psychiatrist with a direct request for couple therapy in order to determine whether her relationship was salvageable. If not, she was clear she would separate but would probably need some support. After three visits, this particular psychiatrist stated it would not be necessary to meet her partner, that she was "a hopeless alcoholic," and that the student herself was "a masochist." He offered to help her "overcome this tendency" but she didn't return.

COMING-OUT PROBLEMS

When women in a lesbian relationship are at different stages of their coming-out process, or are having particular difficulties in evolving through this process, there may be conflict. Often this conflict is based in misunderstanding about the wide gradations in lesbian feeling and responsiveness, and one's self-definition of homosexuality. Sexual orientation is rarely a black-and-white or all-or-nothing phenomenon. Therefore, it is not unusual for two coupled lesbian women to be at different stages of coming out, regardless of their age or experience in the lesbian community. There are almost always misunderstandings about this in those relationships comprised of a woman who has been lesbian as long as she can remember and a woman who was previously married and is still very tentative about loving another woman. In these couples, each partner is anxious—one because she fears abandonment and loss of her partner, the other because she fears loss of her heterosexual and hetero-social identity. This same woman may also have some trepidation and ambivalence about being lesbian, and she may also carry a certain amount of internalized homophobia.

Ann, a family physician, and Catherine, a lawyer, had been together for two years when I first saw them in consultation. Much of their tension and arguing centered around what was termed Catherine's "lack of commitment to the relationship." Individual visits were revealing. Ann was totally un-conflicted about being lesbian, having come out while an undergraduate. She was active in gay and lesbian student groups in college and medical school, volunteered evenings in a downtown gay and lesbian health clinic, and was well integrated into the lesbian community. She had had two previous serious relationships of three-years and five-years' duration, respectively. Catherine, on the other hand, was very unsure of herself regarding her lesbianism. This was her first relationship with a woman, and although her same-sex erotic and loving feelings extended back to adolescence, she never quite trusted them. And they frightened her. She loved Ann deeply and intimately; she really did feel very committed most of the time. What she needed was time and understand-ing. Once Ann accepted this and stopped fearing rejection, their tension and fighting dissipated.

What about the married woman who is involved with another woman before leaving her marriage? These women almost always cite a loss of intimacy with their husbands as a reason for the divorce, that is, loss of emotional and sexual closeness, a sense of leading parallel or divergent lives, a loss of feeling central in their husbands' lives, and so on. There may or may not be a history of same-sex erotic feelings or behavior going back to their adolescent or young adult years. Serendip-itously, these women meet women whom they find interesting, engag-ing, and usually intellectually stimulating. Soon there is a shared sense of intimacy forming; only later does the sexual attraction come into play, and this may be present for some time before being acted upon. Not all of these women become sexual with one another before leaving their marriages. This case is very different from that of married bisexual men who leave their wives for another man.

SEXUAL PROBLEMS

Like heterosexual and gay male couples, lesbians have their share of sexual difficulties. In their monumental study of American couples, Blumstein and Schwartz found that infrequent sexual expression and unequal interest in sex are the commonest complaints in lesbian couples.[14] This has been my clinical impression as well. I would also add that concern about their sexual relationship is never an isolated or solitary complaint or reason for seeking professional help. Either it is one of several complaints or it is viewed by the women themselves as a logical and understandable consequence of not feeling close or not communicating effectively or fighting a lot. This distinguishes them from many heterosexual couples who come with loss of sexual desire or complete sexual absence as a chief complaint and nothing else.

Another difference is the almost universal preservation of nonerotic intimacy in lesbian couples who have not been fully sexual with each other in a long time. What I mean by this is that they continue to be physically affectionate with each other, holding hands, touching, cuddling, hugging, and kissing in a mutually agreeable manner. There seems to be a respectfulness of each other's physical autonomy and rights; there is not the pushing and demandingness for complete genital arousal and orgasm so common in heterosexual and gay male couples. For many lesbian women this intimacy constitutes a comfortable and satisfactory level of sexuality. This behavior may be normative and must be heeded by others, including therapists.[15]

There is a subgroup of lesbian women who have horrendous histories of heterosexual sexual abuse and assault, for example, father–daughter incest, molestation by a male teacher or other adult male, or sexual assault by an acquaintance or date ("date rape"). Some have been raped by strangers; some who have been married before were raped by their husbands. The emotional consequences of sexual abuse and assault are serious and far-ranging. These women have much difficulty trusting others, lack self-confidence, have deep-seated sexual conflicts, feel anxious and phobic, and are subject to mood swings, to name a few sequelae of this type of trauma. Even when they move into a healthy and secure lesbian relationship, some will have much difficulty sexually with their partners. Individual and couple therapy can be very helpful in unearthing and releasing painful memories and feelings with a goal toward a stronger and more confident sense of oneself.

LESBIAN MOTHERS

There are no easily obtainable figures, but a certain number of lesbian physicians have a child or children by a previous marriage, by a consensual arrangement with a selected male friend, or by artificial insemination. Some doctors do not have children themselves but are in a long-standing and committed relationship with another woman with children. These "stepfamilies" are subject to the same sorts of stresses and conflicts as heterosexual stepfamilies but more so, at times, because of the enhanced ambiguities of roles, family secrets, and stigmatization by the rest of society.

A lesbian couple may develop problems if there is a danger or fear of the lesbian mother's not obtaining custody at the time of divorce from her husband or losing custody sometime later. As much as they love and support each other, this stress can be overwhelming if they are isolated from others and do not have adequate personal, familial, and legal support. If the mother's case goes to court, their lesbian relationship becomes public and subject to intense and largely biased scrutiny. Although there are now good studies that document that children reared by lesbian mothers and their partners are at no greater risk for psychiatric illness or gender-identity and sexual-orientation problems than children of heterosexual couples, this information does not easily stand up against the emotionalism and tremendous anxiety in people who are involved in these situations.[16,17] This anxiety is fueled by the often aggressive and blusterous behavior of the newly separated husband and father of the children, whose judgment in seeking legal counsel and solo custody is highly influenced by his monumental hurt and rage over his marriage ending and his wife being with another woman. I would say that this type of separation and divorce is one of the most complicated and distressing types of divorce for doctors and their families.

Another relationship concern that may cause friction between the women is related to the lesbian mother's feeling torn or having loyalties divided between her children and her partner. For example, not all children fully appreciate and understand the precise nature of the relationship between their mother and her "friend." This may be fine for these children, and all they need or want to know. In other households, the relationship is not openly discussed, but the children know. Some children resent their mother's partner not because she is lesbian, but because of other common reasons (they don't want to share her with anyone, they don't want her to get hurt, they fantasize that their parents will get back together, etc.). Other children feel "closeted": they accept their mother's lesbian relationship in the privacy of their home, but they don't share this with their friends; they are afraid and embarrassed to have friends for sleep-overs; and they are subject to ridicule or gossip at school.

These children need to be able to talk about and discuss these feelings with their mother, because they are upsetting and can lead to guilt. Likewise, the mother's partner needs to be able to talk about her feelings of rejection and anger toward the children. A power struggle may develop over the lesbianism itself, with family members becoming polarized and oppositional—one group "politically militant" and the other "politically homophobic." The truth of the situation, of course, lies somewhere in the middle.

SEPARATION PROBLEMS

When a lesbian couple separates, the individuals often do not receive the same amount of consideration and emotional support that is accorded people in heterosexual relationships. This is even more the case if their relationship has been very private and known only to very close friends. The depth of their feeling and intensity of their attachment to each other will be underestimated, even when they have been together for some time. In addition, some people hold cynical and unrealistic ideas about women in lesbian relationships; they believe that their relationships don't last or are fraught with breakups and reconciliations. These are not individuals who will be all that helpful and comforting for lesbian women who are separating.

Making a straightforward and progressive separation from each other may be very difficult for some if not most lesbian couples. Because of issues of fusion that I referred to earlier, plus the sense of mutual caring and engagement women feel toward each other, the actual physical and emotional separation may take some time. There may be resistance to separating on one or both parts; being on one's own again, or for the first time perhaps, is frightening. And if there is a very small local lesbian community there may be fears of never meeting anyone again. However, not all lesbian women who are parting feel this way. Some look forward to being on their own and may remain happily single for the rest of their lives. They derive nurturance and support from their close friends.[18] It is also not unusual for lesbian women who have been coupled at one time to remain life-long friends with each other after the pain of breaking up eases a bit.

Separation is harder and more complicated when there are children. And because there is such ambiguity of roles between the children and their mother's ex-partner during and after separation, plus no legal ties or bonds, issues of values, norms, and responsibilities in both directions are very confusing. When I am involved as a therapist in these types of separations, I do my best to preserve the present and future relationship between the children and the departing noncustodial "parent." They have a right to remain connected and to redefine their situation as the separation evolves regardless of the hurt and anger between their mother and her ex-partner.

Dr. X came to see me on an urgent basis just before separating from Dr. Y, with whom she had been living for twelve years. She was deeply depressed and required medication and twice-a-week supportive psychotherapy visits in the early weeks. Dr. X had three children, all from an earlier marriage, aged fourteen, sixteen, and eighteen. One of her major fears was that Dr. Y would not continue to visit and to be available to her children. Although her former husband had remained involved over the years as the children's father, and they clearly loved and respected him, Dr. X viewed Dr. Y as having been pivotal in their formative years and an essential ancillary parenting figure. Dr. X was doubly anxious about this possible severance of the parent–child relationship because she suspected that Dr. Y was already involved with another woman, who was much younger and had no children. I scheduled an interview with Dr. Y. She loved the children dearly and had no thoughts of not continuing her involvement with them; however, she feared that Dr. X might try to bar access or undermine her relationship with the kids. I then scheduled a visit with the children. Although sad, they had expected their mother and Dr. Y to separate at least two or three years earlier because their relationship had changed so much. They were nervous about their mother's depression and possible self-harm, but they felt confident and secure that they would continue to visit and maintain an ongoing relationship with Dr. Y.

SPECIFIC ISSUES FOR DOCTORS

Up to this point I have been talking about the general psychological and sociocultural stresses for gay male and lesbian couples. What is specific to medical students and doctors? How inhibiting or facilitating are our medical schools and hospitals for gay and lesbian students and doctors? How easy or difficult is it to be openly gay? Are partners of gay and lesbian doctors accorded the same support as wives and husbands of doctors?

Starting with medical school, there continue to be occasional problems with antigay jokes and innuendoes in some lectures or frank bigotry.[19] Most students do not risk speaking up, but some will issue complaints anonymously to the department head or the dean. In some medical schools there is very little teaching on the subject of homosexuality to offset the negatives. During medical school, students are forming and revising their ideas, beliefs, and attitudes on many subjects, homosexuality being only one. They are more sensitive and vulnerable than we like to think. Slanderous and ignorant remarks by faculty not only insult the gay and well-informed students but confuse and taint the poorly informed.

This can be serious. In my role as coordinator of our medical school's clerkship program in psychiatry, I once saw a distraught medical student on an urgent basis two days after a teaching seminar in which the subject of homosexuality was discussed. Several outdated findings that homosexuality is a psychiatric disorder were presented as "facts" by the professor, and disparaging comments were made about the gay student society on campus. This student (an A student) was considering dropping out of medical school because he now wondered if it was possible to be gay and to do a residency! Fortunately, I knew an openly gay resident, and I arranged for them to meet.

Medical school is more than attending classes, clinics, and studying; it also includes participating in and taking advantage of social functions. Most gay and lesbian students will not attend those affairs that are geared toward couples: the annual Medical Ball, graduation dance, and the like. They will probably attend informal get-togethers and parties alone. For some there is a catch-22. If they are closeted, it will be assumed, erroneously, that they are heterosexual; therefore, if they avoid functions, they are deemed antisocial, and if they go alone, they are pressured to bring a date. If they are not closeted, then they and their partners must be prepared to endure the initial awkwardness and perhaps rejection at social events. Attending these events entails making a very powerful and courageous statement that is not only a test of their relationship but also a test of the maturity and integrity of their classmates and faculty. Some students who are especially sensitive make a special and deliberate attempt to ease this process for their gay and lesbian classmates.

Let me turn to residency. Is it any easier to come out to fellow residents than to fellow medical students? Although some gay and lesbian doctors are open about their homosexuality during their residency, most are not. And this is the same throughout their medical careers. It is not just a function of age, maturity, length of time being gay, or being coupled or not. It is largely a matter of personal taste. Many physicians, whether gay, lesbian, or heterosexual, lead private and happy personal lives quite separate from their daily work and their medical associates. They prefer not to socialize with other doctors.

When I talk about gay and lesbian doctors "coming out" or being "open," the reader must remember that these are relative, not absolute, terms. For example, physician A may be open about his homosexuality with his friends, office staff, and physician partners but not the medical community at large or his patients. Physician B may be publicly open to all and also politically committed to gay rights in the local or larger area in which he resides. Physician C may be open to her family and her close friends but no one else. Physicians continue to be held in high esteem in most communities in North America, and these communities vary enormously in their attitudes and beliefs and how they define their respect for doctors. To be openly gay and coupled in San Francisco, California, may actually heighten the favor and regard in which one is held. To be openly gay and coupled in Bakersfield, California, on the other hand, may be suicide, medically speaking.

There are other stresses for gay male and lesbian physicians that affect them personally and that can impinge on their relationship with their partners. Even if they don't break out in "marital symptoms," they may become increasingly insular and isolated as a couple, as described earlier in this chapter, with an "us against them" stance. One of these stresses stems from the mythology about homosexuality, that gay men and lesbian women cannot be trusted with children. Although we physicians see ourselves as intellectually enlightened and unbigoted, there are members of our profession who feel nervous about accepting into a pediatric or child psychiatry residency a gay or lesbian applicant, or reluctant to refer patients to a gay male urologist or lesbian gynecologist. What happens is that gay and lesbian doctors in these fields live in mortal fear that their sexual orientation will be discovered, which, if one stops to think about this for a moment, is a horrible way to live. What is more likely is that they turn away from these specialties during medical school and internship because of these anticipated attitudes and choose something else.

Another stress for gay male and lesbian medical students and doctors is how to get good medical care.[20] They may wonder where they can find a doctor with whom they can be self-disclosing and whom they can fully trust. Usually medical students can obtain this care at the student health center of their university. Even then some students are not certain of confidentiality regarding their medical records and the protection they can expect. By word of mouth, many gay and lesbian medical students and physicians are able to access physicians in the community who are themselves gay or lesbian, or are "gay sensitive."

If they wish to or need to see a psychiatrist, they may worry about whether he or she can accept their homosexuality and, if so, help them individually or as a couple. These worries are superimposed upon all of the usual anxieties and reservations that medical students and physicians have about seeking psychiatric help. This can be overwhelming for some people.

The above comments are most relevant for HIV-positive gay or bisexual male physicians. We know that many studies have shown profound decreases in HIV transmission risk behaviors among gay men, including physicians.[21] We also know that most physicians who are HIV-positive are extremely frightened about disclosure of their illness for many reasons: confusion about contagion, right to privacy (as opposed to the public's right to know), loss of professional livelihood, employer discrimination, threats to insurance coverage, loss of licensure, and economic decline.[22] Some physicians may travel some distance just to ensure some privacy and confidentiality regarding their health care. And all of this occurs in addition to the myriad losses that I discussed earlier.

One final stressor and common problem in today's physicians, irrespective of sexual orientation, is that of competing commitments. In other words, both partners are so busy with their various responsibilities and activities that their relationship suffers in various ways. There may be erosion of relationship solidarity, function, purpose, companionship, and intimacy. Here is an example:

Dr. Green and Dr. Allen were both gay and both were residents. They came for couple therapy because of a sexual complaint—they each had difficulty getting erections and ejaculating when they made love. Without going into detail about the dynamics of their sexual dysfunctions and how I treated them, here are some of the things that were going on in their lives. Dr. Green was in a surgical subspeciality, worked very long days, and was on call at least one day in three. He was on the board of directors of a local art gallery (which consumed a lot of his time), he played in a string quartet, and he volunteered at AIDS Vancouver in his spare time. He was also studying for his fellowship exams, both on his own and in a study group one weekend day a week. Dr. Allen was in a less time-intensive residency, but he did a fair amount of moonlighting to offset fairly substantial education debts and a couple of bad investments. He played baseball, swam on a team, and sang in a choir. He also did volunteer work at a downtown shelter on Sunday mornings and served on a hospital residents' committee. Sadly, he was also HIV-positive, and although he had no symptoms, he was trying to watch the amount of "bad stress" in his life.

In conclusion, gay and lesbian physician couples are more similar than dissimilar to heterosexual physician couples. Like most people, gay and lesbian doctors desire and strive for a close, loving relationship with one particular person—someone who is interested in both individual freedom and personal commitment. I have outlined some of the factors that distinguish these couples from their heterosexual counterparts and give them their unique cast. I have also noted the additional psychological stressors that originate in their belonging to a socially stigmatized minority group.

REFERENCES

1. "Rights Group Backs Homosexual Marriages," *New York Times*, October 28, 1986.
2. Craig R. Dean, "Legalize Gay Marriage," *New York Times*, September 28, 1991, A15.
3. Anna Quindlen, "Evan's Two Moms," *New York Times*, February 5, 1992, A19.
4. Michelangelo Signorile, "Behind the Hate in Oregon," *New York Times*, September 3, 1992, A19.
5. Peter Steinfels, "Beliefs," *New York Times*, September 13, 1992, A18.
6. Joseph H. Pleck, *The Male Myth* (Cambridge: MIT Press, 1981).
7. David McWhirter and Andrew Mattison, *The Male Couple* (Englewood Cliffs, N.J.: Prentice-Hall, 1984).
8. Eli Coleman, "Developmental Stages of the Coming Out Process," in *Homosexuality and Psychotherapy*, ed. John C. Gonsiorek (New York: Haworth Press, 1982), 31–43.
9. Michael F. Myers, *Men and Divorce* (New York: Guilford, 1989), 147–168.
10. Richard C. Friedman, "Couple Therapy with Gay Couples," *Psychiatric Annals* 21 (August 1991), 485–490.
11. Sallyann Roth, "Psychotherapy with Lesbian Couples: Individual Issues, Female Socialization, and the Social Context," *Journal of Marital and Family Therapy* 11 (July 1985), 273–286.
12. Jean Baker Miller, *Toward a New Psychology of Women* (Boston: Beacon Press, 1976).
13. Carol Gilligan, *In a Different Voice: Psychological Theory and Women's Development* (Cambridge, Mass.: Harvard University Press, 1982).
14. Philip Blumstein and Pepper Schwartz, *American Couples* (New York: Williams Morrow, 1983).
15. Martha Kirkpatrick, "Lesbian Couples in Therapy," *Psychiatric Annals* 21 (August 1991), 491–496.
16. Richard Green, "The Best Interest of the Child with a Lesbian Mother," *Bulletin of the AAPL* 10 (January 1982), 7–15.
17. Susan Golombok, Ann Spencer, and Michael Rutter, "Children in Lesbian and Single-Parent Households: Psychosexual and Psychiatric Appraisal," *Journal of Child Psychology and Psychiatry* 24, no. 4 (1983), 551–572.
18. Nanette Gartrell, "The Lesbian as a 'Single' Woman," *American Journal of Psychotherapy* 35 (October 1981), 502–509.
19. Charles R. Fikar, "Mistreatment of Gay Medical Students," *Western Journal of Medicine* 156 (January 1992), 88.
20. David R. Kessler, "The Gay and Lesbian Physician: Unique Experiences, Opportuni-

ties, and Needs," in *The Physician*, ed. J. P. Callan (Norwalk, Conn.: Appleton-Century-Crofts, 1983), 329–351.

21. Deane L. Wolcott, Greer Sullivan, and Dan Klein, "Longitudinal Change in HIV Transmission Risk Behaviors by Gay Male Physicians," *Psychosomatics* 31 (Spring 1990) 159–167.

22. H. D. Scott, "The HIV-Infected Health Care Worker: Another AIDS Policy Conundrum," *Annals of Internal Medicine* 116 (1992), 341–343.

Chapter Five

DIVORCE AND REMARRIAGE

Divorce has become epidemic in North America. Divorce rates have increased fivefold in the past twenty-five years and only now are beginning to level off, and in some years drop slightly. Divorce begins as a psychological process (and I emphasize process—it is not an event) that affects two individuals, that is, the couple who is separating. When there are children, and there are in 50% of divorces, they also become involved in this process. But the impact does not stop here. Parents and grandparents, friends and acquaintances, classmates and workmates, and even neighbors feel its effects. On the Life Stress Events Scale developed by Holmes and Rahe[1] marital separation earns 65 points and divorce 73, surpassed only by the death of a spouse at 100 points.

Divorce is a type of mourning in which the individuals are coming to terms with *loss*—loss of what once was, loss of a happier and more harmonious time, loss of a strong and protective family unit. Some people divorcing are losing contact time with their children, homes, neighbors, friends, and in-laws. Less tangibly, some are losing status, privilege, sameness, predictability, and stability. They may be at various stages of this mourning process—some will deny what is happening, some will be raging, some will be despairing and suicidal, and some will be numb and detached. All will have feelings of failure and variable amounts of self-blame. Like widows and widowers, many will pine for the spouse. This is due to the sense of bonding and attachment that occurs in marriage, especially enduring marriage, and it will be present in those individuals who no longer like, admire, or respect their spouses. One woman said of her ex-husband, a physician, "I can't stand him anymore. I could kill him; his alcoholism has ruined my life. But after twenty-seven years of marriage I can't help but be drawn to him. I'd take him back in a minute if that were possible."

Divorce is painful and symptom producing. Many physicians consult psychiatrists for the first and only time in their lives just prior to or immediately upon separating. Others may not make contact until some months after separating, when divorce is a certainty. "I don't have control over my life" is one of the most common complaints of men and women who are divorcing, and for doctors, who are accustomed to a high degree of control in their lives, this is terribly disconcerting. As time passes some degree of order returns, and a sense of control ensues.

The feelings of failure that accompany divorce are also tough for doctors; for many, this is their first real experience with failing at something in their lives. For those doctors with an exceptionally high drive for accomplishment and excellence, there will also be feelings of shame and guilt for their marriage not succeeding. In fact, they may become quite depressed, and take on more than their share of responsibility for the marriage ending. They may live in the past, obsess over old memories, and berate themselves for not being more involved at home.

One of the most moving experiences for me as a psychiatrist occurred while treating Dr. X, who was at that time head of one of the major departments of a medical school. At his wife's request, they had separated three months before he called me. She had been unhappy for years because of loneliness and emptiness in their marriage. He consistently rejected her entreaties to seek marital therapy, so finally she asked him to leave. At the time of initial consultation, he was quite depressed, experiencing a serious sleep disturbance and suicidal thoughts. He longed for a reconciliation and wanted his wife to come in for marital therapy with him. My single visit with her confirmed my supposition that she was now beyond marital therapy and firm in her desire to remain separated.

Dr. X saw me weekly for several months until he was well again and more adjusted to being on his own. My office became a refuge for this powerful, accomplished, and brilliant man who was seen by most of his peers and all of his residents and medical students as formidable, undaunted, and larger than life. He discussed his inner anguish with no one other than me; in their eyes, he was a rock. Not one of his colleagues ever asked him how he was doing or invited him to talk. I doubt whether he would have opened up, but I'm sure he would have been touched by the gesture. I felt privileged to be able to help him come to terms with his situation and to share his moments of regret, sorrow, and humility. And those moments were profound, for in the naked light of my office, he contrasted his stellar achievements in medicine with the barrenness of his personal being. He vowed to do it differently in his "next life."

What about the frequency of divorce in physicians? Using U.S. census data from 1970 and 1980, Doherty and Burge concluded that both male and female physicians have a lower tendency to divorce than other occupational groups, including other groups of professionals.[2] This is welcome news, in that the common perception among lay and professional groups is that we have higher divorce rates than others. This impression is partly based on publications about troubled medical marriages and partly on longitudinal research,[3] which Doherty and Burge reject as of limited generalizability. I agree with their critical evaluation of the literature regarding the quality and stability of physicians' marriages, but I also agree with Eisenberg that the fact that a marriage lasts tells us relatively little about how good it is.[4] We are wise to remember that divorce rates are only one measure of marital morbidity.

Because there are some gender differences in divorce (men have higher psychiatric morbidity rates[5] and mortality rates[6]), I wish to discuss the issues for male doctors separately from issues for female doctors. There are, of course, many shared concerns and reactions to divorce that are gender free. Also, my division is not intended to be wholly rigid, because of the high number of dual-doctor marriages and the respective problems for each doctor when they divorce.

MALE DOCTORS WHO ARE DIVORCING

MALE DOCTORS WITHOUT CHILDREN

This group of doctors who do not have children are usually but not always younger; some may be older and are childless by choice or have been unable to have children because of infertility. Many of these couples married in medical school or residency. The average length of their marriages is three to five years, and some are agonizing over whether and when to start a family as part of their final demise as a couple. Some of these doctors have been married and divorced before; this divorce may represent a hastily conceived second marriage that has not succeeded.

There is a popular myth that the divorces of childless couples are easier. In practical and legal terms, their divorces are less complicated, but emotionally they are rarely less painful, in some cases more painful. With or without children, people still must deal with their feelings of remorse, anger, guilt, confusion, and apprehension about their future. Unfortunately, the magnitude of this pain is often underestimated by those around them (friends, family, and coworkers) who offer their opinions and advice. Their intentions are good-hearted but their suggestions may be quite inappropriate, or at least premature.

For male physicians, divorce may mean a number of different things, depending upon who initiated the separation. Although the man who leaves his wife may actually feel quite healthy and symptom free at the moment, he did not arrive at that place psychologically without some soul-searching. He will have concluded that his marriage isn't working and that he no longer loves his wife in the way he once did. Despite a calm or cool demeanor, he will feel anxious inside and have many self-doubts: Am I making a mistake in separating? Am I copping out in leaving? Am I too idealistic in my expectations of a marriage partner? Will I ever succeed in love? Am I too selfish, too immature, or narcissistic? Am I too involved in my medical career to give of myself to someone else? These are some of the questions these men may be asking themselves.

It is quite a different picture when wives leave their physician husbands. Elsewhere, I have written about the anger and feelings of abandonment that men experience in general when their wives initiate separation and divorce.[7] Not that women don't feel angry and abandoned when their husbands leave, but their anger takes a different form and they use different coping strategies than men do as a general rule. They are rarely physically violent, and they do not tend to be as isolated as their male counterparts. They more often directly request help and talk about what they are feeling inside.

Some doctors are literally stunned at their wives' decision to leave the marriage. There are feelings of shock, disbelief, and panic. Despite a cognitive awareness of the feelings of unhappiness aired by their wives, they did not realize the gravity of these feelings. As the days and weeks pass, these men are plethoric with emotion: rage one moment and suicidal despair the next; denial of anything amiss today and fear of insanity tomorrow; overwhelming passion for their wives one hour and bitter hatred the next. This reaction was poignantly described by one of my patients, a chief resident in cardiovascular surgery, married five years, who said to me:

> "I'm on an emotional roller coaster. I wake up feeling normal and revved up for work. By the time I get to the hospital I'm tense and furious at her for doing this to me. Then I feel self-righteous and indignant that she would even consider leaving me, let alone actually do it. Next I plot ways of getting back at her, at getting even for the hurt she's caused me. This gives way to guilty feelings, for thinking such cruel and revengeful thoughts. I begin to feel I deserve this and I don't blame her anymore—it's no fun being married to a surgical resident. Then I just feel sad—and empty and terribly alone."

A word about separations that are mutually initiated. It has been my clinical impression that some of these separations are not as mutual as meets the eye. One partner may be much clearer and comfortable than the other, who deep inside is actually feeling quite hurt, or angry, or frightened. However, because of pride or other reasons, this individual needs to maintain a facade of acceptance and self-sufficiency. His or her friends may be fooled by this as well and not be forthcoming or available for support through the divorcing process.

How do male doctors cope with divorce? Is there anything characteristic that is different from other men who are divorcing? Like other men in the professions, doctors may throw themselves into their work in the early weeks and months after separating. Some will date a lot of different women; some will admit that this feels frenetic and not all that satisfying (since AIDS, most men are very careful about their sexual behavior). Many will be aware that they do it to offset feelings of loneliness, that they hate going home to an empty apartment, that they hate cooking and cleaning alone. Because of higher than average earnings, they can choose "the fast lane"—expensive cars, exciting travel, rich furnishings, and lots of personal "toys." Some will drink too much, much more than when they were married, and begin to worry about this. They wonder where it's all heading.

Divorcing doctors differ from divorcing men in the general population when they turn to self-medicating to cope with separation. Of course, self-medication is an occupational hazard for all doctors, but especially so for doctors coping with divorce. Because divorced men have high psychiatric morbidity and mortality rates, they have to be especially careful about their use of tranquilizers and analgesics. I strongly recommend that any separated doctor who takes even one sleeping pill, tranquilizer, antidepressant, or controlled drug from his pharmaceutical samples should consult his personal physician or get an immediate psychiatric opinion on how he's doing.

Men's remarriage rates are higher than those of women, and men also remarry sooner than women do.[8] I don't think that male doctors are any different from men in general, although my statement is totally impressionistic. In most communities, male doctors are still seen as a "good catch" and a welcome commodity in the singles scene. Many divorced doctors know this and find it works both for and against them. Some have difficulty meeting a woman whom they truly trust and respect and with whom they can consider a serious relationship and possible remarriage.

Here is an example of the type of soul-searching that goes on in many individuals before they make a decision to separate:

Dr. K, an epidemiologist, came to see me on his own with this as his chief complaint: "I don't know what I want—I don't know if I want marriage counseling or just out of my marriage. What I do know is that I'm miserable and have been for a long time." He told me that he and his wife had been married for fifteen years and had three children. He was very pent up and spent most of the visit getting a lot of feelings off his chest. In his mind, nothing was working. He gave example after example of unhappy anecdotes of his life with his wife. He felt very demoralized, frustrated, and trapped. One previous attempt at marital therapy two years earlier didn't help.

He had seriously considered separating but balked for several reasons: his wife, his children, his parents (and hers, too), and his fear of failure (he had been married once before). He told me he still loved his wife "but in a different way, like a sister or a good friend. I care about her welfare and her future; I just don't love her in the way I think I should after fifteen years of marriage." They hadn't made love in about six years. They rarely went out together as a couple. Dr. K went on: "I know she must be unhappy, too—but if I bring up separating, I'm afraid she'll go off the deep end. Her parents divorced when she was in high school; I'm not sure she's ever been the same."

Regarding his children, Dr. K described his fears of putting his own children through a separation. He didn't feel that it was fair and that all children deserve an intact home. What he also feared was that his wife, if they separated, might move back to where she grew up and where her mother lived, about a thousand miles away. His close relationship with the children would be over.

Dr. K worried about their respective families' reaction to separation. He and his wife were considered "the model family" of their generation, and because they were both the oldest of their siblings, the fallout would be awful. He was afraid that his father would blame him completely, because he was so fond of Dr. K's wife and saw her as stabilizing. His relationship with his dad had never been easy. He loved his father-in-law more, actually, and anticipated that he would lose him if he and his wife separated. He felt that both his mother and his mother-in-law would understand but "would be heartbroken."

Regarding his previous marriage, Dr. K had agonized a lot when it ended. Although he and his first wife were married only for three years (during medical school) and had no children together, he felt quite ashamed and withdrawn for almost two years, until he met his current wife. He saw himself as a success in many dimensions of his life—especially medicine, athletics, and the piano—but a "complete loser" in marriage.

MALE DOCTORS WITH CHILDREN

With the exception of medical students and residents, most doctors with children who are divorcing are generally a bit older, have been married longer, are at a different stage of their medical career, and are at a different stage of the life cycle. What is ironic is that a large number of these doctors are divorcing just at the time that their workload and their commitment to work are beginning to ease up a bit. In other words, they have finished their residencies, they have secured and expanded a private practice, they have attained a favorable image in the medical community, and their debt load is less severe. Academic physicians will have their research under way, a substantial number of publications, a respected image as a teacher-clinician, and tenure in place. Most will acknowledge that they have devoted an enormous amount of their time and energy to their careers. Only later do they realize that they have paid a very high price; while "making it" their marriages have suffered severely and irreconcilably. This is an example of the "psychology of postponement" in medical marriages so aptly described by Gabbard and Menninger.[9]

Many of these divorces are wife-initiated and for many different reasons. She may feel increasingly estranged and lonely; he may not know what she's talking about, given how busy he is. She may feel it will never get any better, despite his promises and assurances that he's not going to work so hard. She may not love him anymore, except as a family member, in a caretaking way. She may have returned part- or full-time to the paid work force after being home for many years as homemaker, wife, and mother. This work may round out her feelings of self-worth and give her the confidence of "making it" on her own. She may have met another man and, in the throes of this relationship, decided to separate from her husband.

Like the "abandoned" husbands I described earlier, these men may be tremendously distressed. Their rage may become violent and reach a homicidal degree. Their despair may render them helpless and suicidal. As fathers they will be very fearful of losing time with their children and the involvement in their daily lives. They also dread legal intervention and fear being "taken to the cleaners" once the divorce proceedings are under way. Moving into an apartment, no matter how comfortable, is very stressful after being part of a family unit and living in a home for some years. Most of these men are furious and bitter. They felt very disillusioned about how they have led their lives. "All that hard work for this!" is a common lament.

Often these physicians become or attempt to become more involved with their children during and after separation. Sometimes it is too late: Their children are older now and desiring space, divorce or not. Other children flourish with the added paternal time and attention, and usually the physician-father does as well. In fact, most data suggest that those fathers who have continued contact and involvement with their children after separation are less depressed.[10] Further, the father–child relationship during the marriage is not always an accurate predictor of the postseparation relationship: Some men become more active and interested fathers only after separation.[11,12]

There is another group of divorced male doctors who are quite ill, who need treatment but are not getting it. I refer here to physicians who suffer from impairment from alcohol or other forms of drug abuse. These are the physicians who do not seek help voluntarily and are approached by either physician well-being committees or licensing bodies. Some have deteriorated to the point that their medical competence and/or ethics may be suspect.

Let me turn now to the common situation of the male doctor in middle age who leaves his wife and children for another woman, who more often than not is ten to fifteen years younger than the doctor.[13] These are always complicated separations: extremely painful for the wife because she is rejected, upsetting for the man because he is judged harshly, confusing for the children because of divided loyalties toward their mother and father, and upsetting for the new partner who is "the other woman." Rarely does a man just up and leave his wife of many years in an impulsive and callous manner. Usually there have been difficulties for some time but not always openly manifest in the form of tension, arguments, or obvious alienation. There is a conspiracy of silence in some marriages or a neurotic need to keep the peace at all costs; consequently, the normal frustrations and conflicts of marriage never get aired or discussed. Intimacy slowly fades, and the relationship becomes a charade of harmony and normalcy. When the physician enters his middle years, he becomes increasingly conscious of something missing. This feeling of vulnerability is released when he meets someone new who is interested in him. Soon they are seriously involved, emotionally and sexually. With passage of time they, and others, realize that this is not just an affair, but something much more monumental.

There are no easy explanations for this type of separation and why it occurs so frequently. Those who see these middle-aged doctors as scoundrels feel gleeful if these men "pay their dues." Having treated many men married to younger women, I can assure those observers that life isn't always a bed of roses the second time around. There may be sexual concerns as his interest and performance wane with age. There may be sex-role incongruity that leads to marital conflict; for instance, he is old-fashioned and sexist while she is more modern and egalitarian in outlook. She may want children of her own; he must consider becoming an older father, which may necessitate vasectomy reversal. He may be quite threatened by younger men who express passing interest in his wife. He may experience possessiveness, jealousy, and fears of losing her. He may have problems with his children from his first marriage accepting his new wife, and she may have difficulties accepting them. He feels caught in the middle and very torn.

FEMALE DOCTORS WHO ARE DIVORCING

FEMALE DOCTORS WITHOUT CHILDREN

Like male physicians who do not have children, women doctors who are childless and divorcing tend to be younger than their female colleagues with children. However, compared with women in general, this is not the case; like other women with advanced education, women doctors tend to be a bit older when they marry and when they bear children. Some may have been married from five to seven years at the time of divorce.

A feeling of having failed in one's personal life is the greatest issue for a woman doctor going through a divorce. Almost always her career, that is, her professional life, is going very well. Not uncommonly she blames her work and her commitment to it for the failure of her marriage. She may even question, albeit usually only transiently, her whole existence and her choice of medicine as her life's work. In an introspective, obsessive manner, she may become severely self-castigating; she berates herself in a sexist manner for not being at home more, for not cooking more, for not fussing over her husband, for not always acceding to his sexual needs. The more depressed she is, the more there is of this guilty, regretful inner dialogue.

The circumstances of the separation are critical and they will color how she reacts. Those women doctors who initiate their separations will do a lot of this psychological work long before they separate. They may experience a lot of guilt for leaving their husbands but they do not have to come to terms with feelings of rejection (much earlier in their marriages they may have experienced rejection and for this and other reasons, they are now wanting to separate). Those women doctors whose husbands leave them, especially for other women, must work through this feeling of abandonment, loss, and insult to their self-esteem. They will question their femininity, their sense of attractiveness, and their desirability to men—especially if their husband's new partner is younger. The pain can be unbearable and muted only with time.

When Dr. A, a thirty-two-year-old psychiatrist, came to see me her chief complaint was "promiscuity." What she meant by this was that she had been sleeping with several different men over the previous six months. Sometimes these were men she was dating, but not always. Some she picked up in singles bars and took home with her. She was increasingly concerned about her lack of discrimination. Some men were below her in station and frankly dangerous. Others were men she was teaching, a medical student and a psychiatry resident. She acknowledged the fact that she was out of control and that this was atypical behavior for her. Diagnostically, she was quite depressed.

What was significant was that her marriage had ended just before all of this began. Her husband, a surgeon, left her very suddenly. He gave minimal to no explanation for his wish to separate except that "he needed to find himself." Although he denied that there was anyone else in his life, he moved in with a female nurse with whom he worked two weeks after he left Dr. A. Attempts on her part to communicate and to further discuss their separation were rebuffed.

Dr. A had a lot of insight into the dynamics of her situation and did very well with short-term psychotherapy. She knew she was mourning, that she still loved her husband, that she was very hurt and very angry. She was aware that her "promiscuity" was a desperate and inappropriate attempt to regain love and security, to offset feelings of loneliness, and to bolster her shattered self-esteem. Momentarily and fleetingly she felt like a woman again—attractive, desired, and needed. Very soon she was off the treadmill and back in control of her life.

What about the woman doctor who marries a previously married and somewhat older man who already has children by his first marriage? This woman becomes a stepmother at a time in her life when she is ill prepared for this role. She may be in training or just finished. She may have little to no hands-on experience in parenting because of a long commitment to academic pursuits. She has no children of her own. She has a busy career and other responsibilities that her husband may have difficulty appreciating. He may feel she doesn't like his children and resents their weekend and summer vacation visits.

The visitation schedule and custody situation are critical variables here. I have seen many second marriages strained to the point of separation or divorce because of an unexpected and poorly executed change in living arrangements. What I mean by this is that the second wife who starts out as an alternate weekend or summer stepmother suddenly finds herself becoming the primary parent because the biological mother cannot cope, or she relinquishes custody, or the children prefer Dad's home. The physician-stepmother may find herself overburdened and overwhelmed with responsibility. She begins to feel resentful and guilty at the same time. She may worry about the viability of her marriage and begin to abandon her long-standing desire to have children of her own. This makes her even more upset and discouraged. Although feeling hopeless about her marriage, she may fear divorce because she has now bonded with her stepchildren and wonders what kind of relationship, if any, she will have with them after divorce. Indeed, these divorces are very complicated because there are so many parties involved, and very painful because they represent another series of losses for many of the individuals.

Not all women doctors who are childless and unhappy in their marriages will easily opt for divorce. There are many reasons for this, which range from religious and moral dictates (one marries for life, "for better or for worse"), through acknowledging one's dissatisfaction and making the best of a difficult situation, to major fears of being on one's own and possibly single for the remainder of one's life. "I can't understand why she doesn't leave him—she doesn't have children to worry about, she's still young, and she's got a good job and is self-supporting" is a commonly heard statement that does not take these factors into account.

For these doctors, separation and divorce appear frightening and dreary. They do not want to become another divorced-doctor "statistic." They make sweeping generalizations about single or divorced women doctors as "unhappy," "lonely," and "desperate." They recite depressing examples of women doctors they know who never go out, who date "loser after loser," or who throw themselves into medicine "and that's it." Therefore, they debate with themselves whether to remain in their marriages with some of their needs being met or whether to separate and to start afresh.

These are common early concerns for women in unhappy marriages. Fortunately, they do give way to more positive and optimistic ideas about being on one's own after separation. Many women come to a comfortable acceptance of being alone, and may see it as a preferred way to be for themselves. They cherish their independence, their close women friends, and platonic male friends for companionship and shared interests and activities. Some will marry again, some won't. They come to accept the social reality that in the 1990s they, as women doctors, are still a bit of a mystery to most North American men. I say mystery deliberately, because I am trying to avoid concluding that most men are simply intimidated by women doctors. Indeed many are—given the intelligence, the advanced education, the ambition, the status and power, and financial position of women doctors—but I think it is premature and incomplete to generalize at this point in history.

FEMALE DOCTORS WITH CHILDREN

Women physicians who have one or more children generally find their divorces more trying and more complex. As in their marriages, they suffer from role strain—they have responsibilities as doctors (to their patients, students, staff, or colleagues) and as mothers to their children. Depending on their situation, this may mean acquiring and supervising a nanny, or arranging for and transporting children to day care, or securing a day/night babysitter. With older children, divorce may also mean leaving the children unattended after school ("latch-key children") or at night and weekends when called away for emergencies. This may cause worry and guilt. They may also be living on a very tight budget given today's economic climate and student debt load, or if they work only part-time at medicine to have optimal involvement with their children.

All of this is much easier for the woman doctor if she has a communicative, cooperative, and respectful coparenting relationship with her ex-husband. Many do, once the severe hurt and anger of the first post-separation year or two have lessened. These situations, especially the joint custody ones, seem to be the best for all parties—mothers, fathers, and the children. At least they seem the fairest, given the way that parent–child time is divided up, but as of this writing, we do not have good longitudinal research on the long-term mental health implications of joint custody situations for children after divorce.

While on this subject, I wish to mention two observations I have made of women doctors with joint custody arrangements. First, they consistently report a feeling that they are carrying far greater than 50% responsibility for meeting the emotional needs of their children, despite having them for only 50% of the time. This isn't necessarily a complaint on their parts, but more of a gender-specific observation of their role as mothers that transcends marriage into divorce. One woman stated, "My daughter calls me at the office after school every day of the week she lives with her father. We touch base and I hear about any ups and downs that occurred at school. I know she needs this . . . and so do I. She has never been able to talk to her father in this way. He is not interested but denies it."

The second observation is that mothers of young children find it terribly upsetting giving over their children to their ex-husbands for their week as primary parent (i.e., in one-week-on, one-week-off joint custody determinations). Many fathers don't find it easy either, especially if they have been very involved with the children prior to separation. Adjusting to joint custody living certainly takes time; the early weeks and months are the most difficult. Statements like "Not kissing my son goodnight and tucking him in bed at night just kills me" and "Not being there when my daughter's sick in bed with the flu tears me apart, I want to scream" say it all.

Many of these women doctors, especially those with young children, are not interested in meeting new men during the early years of divorce. They find themselves tremendously busy just keeping their heads above water. And if the precipitant for the separation was the husband (e.g., he had repeated affairs during the marriage, or he left her for another woman), she will be so hurt and bitter that she will be completely off men or certainly very cautious. These women find their work, colleagues, children, friends, and hobbies gratifying and sustaining. In fact, they may resent their well-meaning friends pushing them "to go out and meet another man."

Other women, like the childless divorced women doctors I mentioned above, are quite interested in meeting and dating other men but find it frustrating. Either they have difficulty finding men who are stimulating and interesting (and who are unmarried) or they meet only men who seem intimidated by them. Or, because they have children and are already a bit older, they are seen as a liability. Given the contemporary values and norms of mate selection in North American culture, it is easy to see how many of these women never remarry—or choose not to remarry. Unlike men, women doctors are more likely to have a supportive network of friends and family while going through divorce. They are also more willing than their male counterparts to take advantage of professional help for emotional support and guidelines about the divorcing process as they progress through it.

Like women in general, there are a significant number of women physicians whose marriages end and who manage very well on their own. In addition to adjusting to their own personal hurt and loss, many of these women are helping their children cope with the family breakup. This "behind-the-scenes" work is illustrated in the following example. I never actually met Dr. X, only her husband, who was my patient:[14]

Mr. X, a fifty-two-year-old bank manager, came to see me three months after he had separated from his wife. He told me that he had a lot of mixed feelings about being separated and wondered: "Is this normal?" He and his wife had been married for twenty-eight years, having met as college students, and they had five children ranging in age from twenty-five to fifteen years old. He said that he had been unhappy in his marriage for many years but that he never considered separation because he was Catholic and because he had always felt that divorce was a selfish act, "great for the parents, cruel for the children." Two years before he left his wife, he met another woman, Mary, and they became "just friends" for many months. They didn't see each other often because she lived and worked in a nearby city. However, they gradually became more intimately, and sexually, involved. Quite naturally, Mr. X was then forced to make a decision; after several months of soul-searching, contemplation, and consultation with his parish priest, he decided to leave his marriage.

When I asked Mr. X how his wife and the children were handling the separation, he told me that his wife was a "brick." "She's been very understanding and brave; I know she feels humiliated inside. I'd feel better if she'd get angry at me, or if she hated me, but she doesn't." His children were divided, along age lines, about the separation—the three older children were somewhat detached about it and felt that their parents just had to do what was best for each of them. His oldest son told Mr. X that he was surprised that his father hadn't left ten years earlier. The fifteen-year-old and seventeen-year-old, both girls, were very upset about the separation and were both angry at him. They made frequent excuses not to see him and often canceled scheduled plans they had made to do something with their father. They both admitted to their father that they might have been more "forgiving" if there weren't another woman, "especially someone fifteen years younger than Mom."

Mr. X, initially relieved and excited to have made the decision to separate, began to feel increasingly guilty as the weeks and months went by. He was no longer enjoying his relationship with Mary and now felt guilty about that. Ideas of reconciling became increasingly urgent, and he began discussing this with his wife. They went out a couple of times: "the first time it was wonderful; the second time it was horrible." Mary became threatened and worried about this, and she decided to pull back from the relationship. About this time, Mr. X also found it hard to do his work as efficiently and conscientiously as he normally did. He was preoccupied and forgetful; he developed early morning dread and wakefulness. He lost his appetite. He agreed to take an antidepressant, which helped him to begin to cope again. His guilt lessened, and he was able to feel more confident in his decision making. He abandoned his notions of reconciling. After a few weeks, he had a frank and open talk with his teenage daughters, and they began to warm up to him a bit. Eventually he and his wife divorced.

CHILDREN OF DIVORCING DOCTORS

I would like to leave the issues of divorce for male doctors and female doctors, and turn to the children. What are their concerns? Can anything specific be said about them in addition to what is known about children in general whose parents are divorcing or divorced? First of all, they are all middle- to upper-middle-class children. Their standard of living will decrease somewhat or a lot in accordance with the divorce settlement, the amount of the child support payments, and if the latter are rigorously met. Much will depend upon whether their father, mother, or both are doctors and whether their mother, father, or both have custody. The greatest decline in living standard occurs in male physician marriages designed along traditional lines with wives home full-time with young children. These women are usually less educated than their physician-husbands. When they attempt to reenter the paid work force after divorce, their skills may be outdated, they need retraining, and even then may not earn very much relative to their former husbands' income. In general, divorced ex-wives of doctors have much lower standards of living than their remarried ex-husbands. This can cause resentment and jealousy.

Some children of divorced doctors harbor negative feelings toward the physician-parent(s). These are not uncommon in children of divorce and are rooted in loss—loss of the family unit, loss of an idealized notion of the family, loss of time with one or both parents, loss of nurturing and attention by one or both parents. But children of doctors are sometimes struggling with a particular type of negative feeling that may be confusing for them and also cause them to feel guilty. What I am referring to here is the situation in which there is a marked discrepancy between the physician's public image and his or her personal or family image. I will use the divorced male physician as the prototype. If his children do not have a clear empathic understanding of the divorce and if he does not cultivate and preserve a strong, caring, and predictable relationship with them, these children will become resentful. They will feel shortchanged and unloved. But because he is a doctor and all that this conjures up (hardworking, busy, dedicated, respected, accomplished, etc.), they may feel ashamed of their feelings. Not all children are as clear and articulate as one twelve-year-old boy who said to me, "My dad may be a wonderful doctor, but he's a loser of a father."

There is a greater risk of an unhealthy adaptation to divorce if the physician-father overworks and underestimates the psychological needs of his children. These needs are especially important during the early weeks and months after separation, when children are the most vulnerable. Ironically some physician-fathers throw themselves into their work at this time in order to cope with their pain at not seeing their children on a daily basis, when their wives have custody. Both fathers and the children may feel angry and rejected; and if these men move quickly into new and serious relationships with other women, these feelings may be compounded.

I will briefly sketch a not uncommon portrait of events when this situation occurs. The new relationship may progress rapidly, and soon the physician and his new woman friend are living together. Some time for adjustment is required as the children come to know and begin to like "Dad's new girlfriend" and she comes to know and accept them. Meanwhile, depending on the time interval and acuteness of the separation, the children's mother will need time to adjust to their being "exposed" to this woman. She may be angry that her former husband no longer sees the children on his own, that this new person is present, that the children have to share him with her. She may also feel personally threatened by this woman's new role in her children's lives. If she still loves her former husband or has unresolved feelings about the divorce, she may feel furious and ripped apart inside at the creation of a new family unit at her ex-husband's home. This cannot help but be felt by the children, who feel awkward and torn. At this point, they become cautious, guarded, and reluctant to report events in each household to the opposite parent.

If the man's relationship leads quickly to remarriage and children, this may set off another turn of events. He may work even harder now because he is supporting a new family plus paying child support (and possibly alimony) to the first. He gets weary and resentful, and so may his second wife. The children from his first marriage feel "shoved aside" by his second family, or at least lower down on his list of priorities. Although they are now older, perhaps teenagers, they are no less in need of his continued love, guidance, discipline, and companionship. Their mother may also feel bereft of his assistance and investment as a coparent; this can become intense for her, especially if the children begin to have problems. Commonly, if she has not remarried she will not have the love and support of a husband and stepfather.

I want to turn now to the children of dual career, coprofessional couples who are divorcing. Never in the history of North America have there been so many couples who both have careers and are striving for egalitarian principles in the design of their marriages. Many of these divorcing professionals have one or more children. In many of these divorcing professional couples, both are doctors.

What I have noticed in my practice is a movement toward historically conventional sex roles at the time of and during the early stages of the divorce. In other words, it is the female professional who cuts back on her work outside the home to spend more time with the children and to get established or become adjusted to being on her own. Her activities may include arranging meetings with realtors, lawyers, accountants, teachers, and therapists. Their husbands, on the other hand, may work harder, partly for financial reasons (they begin to realize the enormous cost of divorce) and partly for the psychological reasons described earlier. As time passes and both can see their way clearly, commitment to their careers and to their shared children becomes more balanced.

When two professionals divorce each other, there is a risk of over-gratification of their childrens' material needs. Both are high wage earn-ers and can afford it. If they are very busy with their careers, they may feel guilty that they do not have a lot of time to spend with the children; they may unconsciously compensate with material goods. They may also feel guilty about the marriage breaking up and feel sorry for the children; this may lead them to overspend and overgratify. Most professionals are perfectionists. With perfectionism comes guilt and a sense of personal failure when ideals are not met or maintained. They may have difficulty setting limits and be very inconsistent with their discipline. Soon these overindulged children are playing off their divorced parents. They become omnipotent and develop an attitude of entitlement.

This situation can become even more serious if each parent is en-gaged in some type of competitive power struggle to outdo the other in providing for the children. This can happen if they are both angry at each other for the divorce, greatly mistrust the other, and vie for the children's love through gratification. Each rationalize it as "want-ing the best for my children," but there are consequences. I once as-sessed two young children, aged seven and ten, whose parents had been separated about one year. Their father was an ophthalmologist, their mother a radiologist. These children had two sets of everything, one in each home—every conceivable toy and game, bikes, skis and ski outfits, tennis rackets, personal computers, and the like. They dressed only in designer clothes. Every weekend was a flurry of activity: skiing with mother one weekend, sailing with father the next, or hiking, or riding, or taking unending lessons. They had traveled to more vacation spots in their short lives than most people do in a lifetime. They had little say in all of this; their main complaint was that they got tired "some of the time."

Many dual-career couples who divorce have a joint custody ar-rangement for the children. This arrangement usually means equal time in each household but not always; joint custody may be shared rights and decision making only. One of the homes, usually mother's, is the principal residence for the children, who see their father only on week-ends, every other weekend, or according to whatever visitation schedule has been mutually arranged. My clinical experience with couples who share their children equally, say one week at Dad's and the next week at Mom's, has been that it is well received and favored by the parents. This is supported by the literature on divorce. As I mentioned earlier, we do not yet have extended research on the children.

WHY DO DOCTORS DIVORCE?

I think that the best answer to this question is another question: "Why do people divorce?" We know that there are sociological and psychological factors that contribute to marital breakdown and divorce as we move from general and impersonal factors to those that are more specific and personal. If we ask another question—"Why don't all people with marital breakdown divorce?"—I can begin to speculate about doctors and divorce.

First, most doctors can afford to divorce. At first this sounds like a very superficial reason for ending a marriage, but it is not meant to be inane. Divorce is an expensive process when one begins to consider costs of legal fees, accountants, therapists, mediators, establishing and maintaining a second household, moving expenses, duplication of some possessions, child support, and maintenance. Not all couples have expenses in all these areas, but certainly in some. Financial possibility is not necessarily a conscious and deliberate reason to divorce, either; it is always coupled with serious marital unhappiness.

Having the financial means (or the prospect of these means) is an extremely important facilitating factor for unhappily married women medical students and physicians who wish to leave their marriages. Financial well-being, along with their job security, confidence, and ambition, gives them a greater measure of assurance that they can make it on their own. When they have children, this assurance is even more critical. One can really appreciate the power of money and its ability to buy freedom, independence, and sometimes safety when one treats married women and mothers who are poor and are in desperately unhappy and dangerous relationships. For in these marriages, the women not only lack a clear sense of themselves as capable and competent persons but also lack the financial resources to get out and get started.

Another observation about doctors that might contribute to their ability to consider divorce as a solution to marital unhappiness is that they are accustomed to taking charge, to problem solving, to trying to make things better, to being in control. Being unhappily married is rarely a pleasant feeling; it makes you tense, or depressed, or spills over into your work. Also, because some physicians (those in family medicine, psychiatry, or internal medicine) are confronted daily with a range of life's vicissitudes in their offices, they do not view divorce as shameful or frivolous. They see its necessity in many marriages and the resultant happiness in one or both partners after the initial upset. They come to see that there is possibility and hope for themselves in ending their own miserable and no longer viable marriages.

How did they get there in the first place? Why are they or their spouses so unhappy? Again there are no easy answers to these questions, but allow me two observations that I see commonly in my office: first, these doctors work too hard and neglect their spouses and children; and second, they do not communicate very well in their marriages. For some doctors, these problems are connected: the harder they work, the less they communicate at home, and vice versa, the harder they find it to communicate at home, the more they work.

Let me elaborate a bit. Most physicians are not strangers to hard work. For many it began in childhood, in working hard either physically or academically or both. Many physicians have come from homes with hardworking parents as role models. College, medical school, internship, and residency reward and reinforce this propensity and capacity in doctors. Once doctors are established in clinical practice or its academic and administrative equivalent there is always work and more work available. It can become galvanizing and magnetic in its pull.

Hard work, especially medical work, is ennobling in our society. And herein lies a contradiction for some doctors. Their work may begin to compensate for their liabilities (both real and imagined) as husbands and fathers, as wives and mothers. It becomes easier to work late, to see more patients, to write more papers, to take on more committee work than to learn to communicate more effectively and more intimately at home. Once problems arise at home, work really becomes attractive, demanding, and imperative. Soon the doctor is on such a treadmill that it is very hard to jump off.

With regard to communication in marriage, no one is born with an inherent ability to succeed easily here. All married people have difficulty making their needs, wishes, and complaints clear and comprehensible to their spouses. Improving communications involves making the time and having the desire to do so, having the courage to take risks in being open, having the maturity to accept the honesty of one's spouse, and making one's marriage a priority. As a group, physicians are probably no better or no worse than any others at communicating. But we don't win any prizes, either. Patients continue to complain about the lack of "humanism" in their encounters with doctors. We are trained and expected to be "clinically objective" in our work. In some branches of medicine, we "process" an enormous amount of emotionally disturbing events in the course of a working day. Are we being numbed by it all? Do we carry this numbness into our other lives as spouses and parents? Do we carry the politics of the workplace, which can be considerable and require "strategies," that is, caution, intellectual astuteness, manipulation, bargaining, and cool control, into our marriages?

While they are divorcing, doctors must continue with the everyday responsibilities of their lives, all of which might be quite substantial. I am amazed at the number of doctors I see who continue to work full-time through a divorce. This is more so for male doctors; female doctors, especially mothers, allow themselves more personal time to heal and to tend to their children's needs. Many doctors are on "automatic pilot" during the early weeks and months after separation, but this is what works for them. This coping strategy has often served them well in the past in times of crisis and turmoil. One obstetrician said to me, "Actually, I'm going through the motions of living. I'm working just as hard and just as competently as ever, but I'm not there. I'm concentrating OK and my judgment is fine; that doesn't worry me. But my friendliness at work is all an act. This is the same way I got through my mother's death when I was in medical school."

In addition, work is therapeutic for most people. It does enable them to put their troubles aside, fully or partially, for several hours each day. Some physicians will not be able to work for a few weeks because they are too symptomatic. They may be depressed or anxious, have a sleep disturbance or loss of appetite, or be unable to do their work without breaking down. Taking sick leave, including medical disability for a few weeks, plus consulting a physician become essential. This person can then provide the support and direction that the physician-patient temporarily needs.

Practicing medicine when one is not feeling well is ill-advised; it is not fair to oneself and certainly unfair and possibly dangerous to the patient. Patients have the right to expect their doctors to be alert, conscientious, and empathic. Further, we have an ethical obligation to provide competent care. Some patients who come in with marital and divorce problems will unknowingly upset their physicians because the concerns are so close to home. It is very hard to help others when one's own wounds are so fresh.

How long does it take to get over a divorce? Responses to this question range from "a few months" to "you never get over it." There are many variables, but most people do not begin to feel back on their feet, so to speak, for at least a year. By three to five years most people can make the following statements: "I'm back in control of my life again"; "I can now talk about my divorce without crying"; "I can finally get on with my life again"; "The bitterness is gone now"; "I've stopped wanting to kill her (him)"; "It was horrible—I'm a different person now than I was then."

DOCTORS AND REMARRIAGE

In the United States, 80% of divorced people remarry, and of all people marrying for the first time, 19.5% marry a divorced person.[15] As I mentioned earlier, men remarry more quickly than women and at a higher rate. There is now some evidence that the incidence of redivorce is increasing, especially in younger people, with as many as 20% of all individuals now in their thirties expected to eventually divorce twice.[16] A study of male physicians who had divorced more than once revealed that they exhibited greater nonconforming, impulsive, and risk-taking tendencies than both never-divorced and once-divorced physicians.[17]

Let me elaborate on this a little. Not only do people who are impulsive leave their marriages somewhat abruptly, but they also move quickly into new relationships. Some of these relationships have started prior to separation from the spouse. There may be little to no courtship or time to get to know the person before they are living together or getting married. There may be unresolved issues from the earlier marriage that have not been settled, like financial concerns, division of assets, and regular and predictable visitation of the children, to say nothing of the emotional aspects—coming to terms with loss, persistent feelings of care and attachment to the former spouse, as well as feelings of failure, anger, and the like. Some of these individuals have never lived on their own or have never been without a special person in their life; consequently, there is always a flurry of activity and energy investment to ward off feelings of loneliness, despondency, or panic. A vicious circle is set up, because their anxiety or impulsivity leads to a poor choice of mate. This choice puts them at further risk for relationship conflict and breakdown. Also, if they get bored easily, they will not be able to accept and understand the routinization characteristic of all marriages.

With regard to forming stepfamilies, I have already mentioned the difficulties that can arise for the childless woman doctor who becomes a stepmother. Much the same can occur for the male physician who has no children of his own when he becomes a stepfather, especially in the areas of financial and emotional responsibility. Most often he has had no experience whatsoever as a parenting figure; his age and maturity, plus the ages of his stepchildren when he enters their lives, are significant variables. He must be especially careful not to rush into having children of his own with his new wife. There is a serious risk of never completely bonding with his stepchildren, so that he and they lack a secure foundation that they can all count on before a new family is conceived. What develops is a stepfamily that lacks solidarity and cohesion—there are splits and cracks, family subsystems, and a lot of unhappy people who feel unloved.

While I'm on the subject of stepfamilies, one must never forget the influence of the families of origin of each adult as well as the families of origin of their ex-spouses. I am referring here to all of the extended family—mothers-in-law, fathers-in-law, sisters-in-law, brothers-in-law, aunts, and uncles from their previous marriage(s). In the typical remarriage of two people who have both been married before, and who both bring children into this marriage, we are talking about an enormous number of people, all with a varying intergenerational connection to this new family. Because there are no precedents for this phenomenon in the history of North America, there are no rules, no guidelines, no norms. It is easy to appreciate why there may be friction if Kristin's paternal grandmother from her mother's first marriage wants to see her at Christmas, but she is already committed to visiting her maternal grandmother and her new stepbrother's grandmother!

Earlier I discussed some of the concerns of children when their divorced physician-father remarries and starts another family. What about the man himself? What are the risks for him? He may get on a treadmill of work, work, and more work. Agewise he is probably in his peak years. He not only has an established reputation in the community but also finds work very compelling and gratifying. His hospital committee and community work may increase at the same time. Expenses increase commensurate with his high income. Soon he is working nonstop. This, coupled with genetic predisposition and other factors, may put him at risk for a coronary or hypertension. Emotionally he may begin to feel burnout or symptoms of depression. His consumption of alcohol or his use of sleeping medication may increase. His second marriage may begin to founder.

Remarried male physicians who reach this point or worse are not common. Most doctors in a second marriage are tuned in to the early warning signals of working too hard or marital difficulty. Because they are older and more mature at the time of this marriage, they already have a greater capacity for reflective decision making about whom they marry and a better understanding of marital expectations and responsibilities as the result of an earlier marriage. They have usually learned a lot about themselves through the ups and downs of the first marriage and through the process of divorce. They communicate more effectively and love more selflessly. Some lead quite a different, simpler life-style—they don't work as hard, live on less income, and relax more. If problems do arise that they and their wives cannot solve, they are more amenable to seeking marital therapy than they were in their first marriage.

Divorced women doctors, with or without children, do not marry again at the same rate as their male physician colleagues. For many this is fine. They are happy with their careers, their homes, children (if they have children), friends, and extended family. They enjoy the independence and freedom to pursue interests and hobbies and travel as they like. Some have short-term relationships that are satisfactory and a source of contentment. Remarriage is not completely ruled out, but it does not figure in their short-term plans or goals. "Maybe when my children are off to college, I'll give it a whirl—right now I have enough on my plate" was said half-jokingly but also seriously by one of my patients, an oncologist with two teenagers.

Like most divorced people, women doctors may be wary and show customary fearfulness about embarking on a second marriage. And this wariness will be highly colored by the dynamics of the first marriage and the problems that contributed to its breakdown. In the early stages of a new relationship with a man, the woman physician will watch for warning signals reminiscent of the first marriage: Am I getting involved too quickly? Is he? Am I beginning to lose my independence? My assertiveness? My self-respect? My identity? Is he strong enough for me? Does he drink too much? How trustworthy is he? How much does he understand and appreciate the nature and importance of my work?

There is the added guardedness about the man's motives and intent, which I have noted in some divorced women doctors involved in new relationships. More specifically, she becomes aware that she is well set up and established—she has her own home, nice furnishings, a good income, job security, and status. She may have a nice circle of friends, many of whom are financially comfortable, or interesting, or know how to live well. She knows that she is bright, a hard worker, and responsible. If events in this relationship cause her to doubt her boyfriend's sincerity as an accomplished person in his own right, or his potential if he is in an early phase of his career, she will become cautious. She may also fear exploitation, especially if he bristles at the thought of a prenuptial agreement or marriage contract.

Dr. A realized this too late, and her realization precipitated her coming to see me one month after her hastily conceived second marriage. She was very distraught and in terrible conflict. On her honeymoon she had begun to feel that her new husband was deceiving her with regard to his financial resources, both at present and in the recent past. He had omitted many important details during their courtship that, in retrospect, seemed fundamental. When they returned from the honeymoon, she made some phone calls that confirmed her worst fears. Her trust was gone; she became frightened, angry, and avoidant. Her husband's redeeming features, the major features that she had fallen in love with, were now overshadowed by this massive subterfuge. They separated six weeks after marriage.

CONCLUSION

In this chapter I have discussed many of the characteristics of the divorcing process and its impact on men, women, and their children. I have identified some of the determinants specific to male and female doctors. There are gender contrasts that affect the dynamics of the separation itself—before, during, and after. Indeed, men and women do separate differently. Divorce remains a complicated process. Always emotionally unsettling, it is more upsetting for some, less upsetting for others. Time is the best healer, with or without remarriage.

REFERENCES

1. T. Holmes, "Life Situations, Emotions, and Disease," *Journal of the Academy of Psychosomatic Medicine* 19 (December 1978), 747–754.
2. William J. Doherty and Sandra K. Burge, "Divorce Among Physicians: Comparisons with Other Groups," *Journal of the American Medical Association* 261 (April 28, 1989), 2374–2377.
3. George E. Vaillant, N. C. Sobowale, and C. McArthur, "Some Psychological Vulnerabilities of Physicians," *New England Journal of Medicine* 287 (1972), 372–375.
4. Leon Eisenberg, "Marriage: If It Lasts, Does That Mean It's Good?" *Journal of the American Medical Association* 261 (April 28, 1989), 2401.
5. W. Gove, "The Relationship between Sex Roles, Marital Status, and Mental Illness," *Social Forces* 51 (December 1972), 238–244.
6. W. Gove, "Sex, Marital Status, and Mortality," *American Journal of Sociology* 79 (July 1973), 45–67.
7. Michael F. Myers, "Angry Abandoned Husbands: Assessment and Treatment," in *Men's Changing Roles in the Family,* ed. Robert A. Lewis and Marvin B. Sussman (New York: Haworth Press, 1986), 31–42.
8. H. Ross and I. Sawhill, *Time of Transition: The Growth of Families Headed by Women* (Washington, D.C.: Urban Institute, 1975).
9. Glen O. Gabbard and Roy W. Menninger, "The Psychology of Postponement in the Medical Marriage," *Journal of the American Medical Association* 261 (April 28, 1989), 2378–2381.
10. John W. Jacobs, "The Effect of Divorce on Fathers: An Overview of the Literature," *American Journal of Psychiatry* 139 (October 1982), 1235–1241.
11. M. E. Hetherington, M. Cox, and R. Cox, "Divorced Fathers," *Family Coordinator* 25 (1976), 417–428.
12. Judith S. Wallerstein and Joan B. Kelly, "Effects of Divorce on the Visiting Father–Child Relationship," *American Journal of Psychiatry* 137 (December 1980), 1534–1539.
13. Michael F. Myers, *Men and Divorce* (New York: Guilford, 1989), 94–110.

14. Ibid., 201–202.
15. Ira D. Glick and Oliver Bjorksten, "New Demographic Trends in American Marriage," paper presented at the American Psychiatric Association Meeting, May 10, 1984, Los Angeles.
16. Paul C. Glick, "Marriage, Divorce, and Living Arrangements: Prospective Changes," *Journal of Family Issues* 5 (1984), 7–26.
17. Edward W. McCranie and Joel Kahan, "Personality and Multiple Divorce," *Journal of Nervous and Mental Disease* 174 (March 1986), 161–164.

Chapter Six

OLDER PHYSICIANS AND THEIR MARRIAGES

In this chapter I want to discuss common themes and conflicts for physicians who are approaching their sixties or are in them. This is a stage of life when humans are trying to deal effectively with aging, illness, and death while simultaneously retaining a zest for life.[1] As married individuals, their task is to support each other in their struggles for fulfillment and productivity in the face of aging. They try to remain intimate with each other despite fears of sexual failure, desertion (by death or divorce), and loneliness. Often both partners are grappling with loss as family members and close friends move away or die. One's physical surroundings also change if there is a move from the family home into an apartment or from a diverse residential neighborhood into a retirement community.

Ageism (i.e., a discriminatory attitude toward older people) is very real in North American society. Yet this phenomenon is not well understood or respected. As a clinician, I am not qualified to give an analysis of ageism's origins, manifestations, pervasiveness, and politics, but I am certain of one thing: being judged or treated unfairly because one is becoming older is a significant stressor for people and affects their mental health.

When we consider the older physician and his or her family, we are usually thinking, albeit narrowly, of two people. Usually their children have grown and are living on their own, married, or in some other committed relationship. There may or may not be grandchildren who live near or far. Therefore, for most of the time, the physician's family is now very small. And this can feel lonely, boring, and rather depressing. Many older physician couples do not fit the stereotype promulgated by the advertising industry in banking or investment ads or travel brochures of the attractive older couple with lots of gray hair, big smiles, and porcelain-white teeth as they head off to the golf links or tennis courts together!

RETIREMENT ISSUES

With increasing longevity, many physicians are living longer and, if their health permits, practicing medicine long past the common retirement age of sixty-five years. This can present a type of marital problem that is based in incongruous expectations of one another at this stage of the marital life cycle. For example, if the physician is a man and has been working hard for many years, his wife may have expected that they would have more time together in these years—time to take up leisure activities, spend with grandchildren, travel, and so forth. If the physician is a woman, her husband may have had similar expectations of more time together. These spouses then may feel lonely and resentful that they have "sacrificed" many good years with nothing forthcoming in return.

Dr. S and Dr. W were both physicians and both seventy-five years old. They came to see me in a crisis because Dr. W had threatened to leave her husband unless he retired. They were both family physicians and had practiced together until Dr. W retired at sixty-five years of age. She stopped work because she was well and wanted to do many things in life that she had never had time to do previously because of her work schedule. After ten years of fulfilling many of her plans, she now wanted to travel. It was her understanding that her husband had wanted to do the same and, furthermore, that he had promised he would retire when he was seventy.

Dr. S really didn't have much of a defense. He did not deny that he wanted to travel and saw that in their future plans, nor did he deny that he had planned to retire when he turned seventy. "I just love medicine," "I love my patients; who will look after them if I retire?" "The years pass so quickly; am I really seventy-five?" and "I guess I figure I'll live forever, and we can always travel later" were some of Dr. S's statements as he mused aloud in my office.

Over the course of three appointments and much reassuring discussion about his responsibilities to his patients and their welfare, Dr. S. began to wind down his practice. He found a younger doctor to take over his remaining patients, and he fully retired three months later. Shortly thereafter, I received a postcard from Dr. W and Dr. S from Australia, the first leg of a four-month South Pacific journey. They were having a lot of well-deserved fun together.

Another problem that may arise around retirement occurs when or if the physician and his or her spouse decide to sell their home and move away, often to a warmer climate or to a retirement community. It may not work out for several reasons. Sometimes they find that they are much younger (both chronologically and psychologically) than their neighbors. Or they may be bored despite a smorgasbord of available leisure activities in their community. Or they may miss their long-standing friends or family members. Or the physician may miss practicing medicine and feels bereft of the many needs that were being met by looking after patients. If this feeling does not end after several months of trying to adjust to retirement, the physician may need to consider some form of work, medical or otherwise, in order to begin to feel happy and fulfilled again.

There is a huge difference between voluntary and forced retirement. Physicians who retire from medical practice, teaching, or administration completely of their own accord are usually psychologically ready. They have been considering this for some time and may have even semiretired or begun to do less paid work and pursue avocations and so forth. When forced retirement occurs because of institutional policy (e.g., everyone retires on or before their sixty-fifth birthday), licensing regulations, or failing health, many practitioners are not happy about it, no matter how much forethought has transpired. In fact, many are angry, and some fight it, successfully or unsuccessfully. And some develop symptoms of a psychiatric illness and/or marital strain during or as a consequence of this assault to their professional equilibrium and livelihood.

Dr. P was referred to me by his internist for "paranoia." The background was as follows: Dr. P was an academic pathologist who had retired from the medical school where he had worked for thirty years. This was one year before I was asked to see him in consultation. Three months into his retirement, Dr. P developed diabetes, and this was very distressing for him. He didn't cooperate well with dietary restrictions, blood glucose monitoring, or taking his insulin. He yelled at his wife and berated her when she tried to discuss her concerns about his health. He was withdrawing more and more into his study to complete a number of scientific articles based on his research that were not completed by the time he retired. He was losing weight and not sleeping. Mrs. P called her husband's internist and requested a psychiatric consultation the day after their son's wedding—Dr. P refused to attend the wedding because he had "too much work to do!"

Dr. P was quite willing to see me, but he insisted there was nothing wrong with him. He explained: "At least you're willing to listen to me—everyone else I talk to thinks I'm nuts. I've been pushed out of the university by a bunch of nitwits. No one in the department understands my outstanding credentials and my scholarly record. Do you know how many articles I've written? How many books? I'm world famous, and none of my colleagues will ever attain one tenth of what I've accomplished. Do you know how much grant money I secured the past five years? Do you know how many pathologists I've recruited the past ten years? Who put this rinky-dink backwater of a pathology department on the map? They're all a bunch of goons, and they've conspired and plotted to get me out. They say it's my age, but that's hogwash. I'm as mentally fit as a thirty-year-old."

I was able to conduct a thorough assessment of Dr. P's mental functioning and I found him to be very depressed, but not suicidal. His attention span and ability to concentrate were poor. Despite hours in his study daily, he was making no progress with his scientific papers. He did have a lot of paranoid thoughts. He was willing to take an antidepressant medicine and return for supportive psychotherapy, on his own and with his wife. He responded nicely, and within a month was much better and had a more realistic understanding of retirement. For several sessions, he was able to talk about what his career had meant to him, how much his self-esteem depended on it, how awkward he felt outside of his "work role," how distant he felt from his wife and kids, how inadequate he felt as a man, and how guilty he felt if he was not working twelve or more hours a day!

This case example touches on an issue that may be a conflict for retiring physicians, especially male physicians, and that is dependency. Aging renders us more dependent upon others, and this can be tremendously upsetting for men who have taken pride in being self-sufficient and in control throughout their lives. Given how physicians are masters at denial, it is not uncommon for aging physicians to deny their dependency on others or to fight it continually with behaviors that are unpleasant, stubborn, or obstructionistic to those around them.

LOSS

Another type of marital problem has to do with loss. As we age, loss is an ever-present companion. There may be sudden or gradual loss of health that can result in restricted mobility because of body weakening, visual or auditory impairment, or inability to drive a motor vehicle. This loss of physical vitality and livelihood can make people feel despondent as their worlds become more restricted and programmed. Marital life may become dull and boring, or tension filled, if individuals take their personal frustrations and forced dependencies out on each other.

Most aging couples, medical or not, worry about finances and living on a fixed income. And this is even more manifest during times of economic recession and inflation. Again, if one worries more than the other and is reluctant to spend money, the spouse may feel trapped and unhappy. Life begins to feel like an endurance test or a waiting game— waiting to die.

Dr. and Mrs. I were referred to me by Mrs. I's family physician, who was convinced that her many hypochondriacal symptoms were related to marital unhappiness. When I met the two of them in my office, it was Dr. I who stated that he would love to do more things with his wife if only she were physically able. Mrs. I argued that it was not her health at all but her husband's "stinginess" with money that precluded their going out to restaurants, visiting their children and grandchildren (who lived about a thousand miles away), or taking midwinter "warm weather" vacations. She told him she would feel instantly better if he planned an evening out together or booked a trip.

What I discovered on closer examination of Dr. I was that he was actually quite depressed and that his worry about money, although not delusional, was certainly excessive given their resources. Further, this was only one symptom—he had also become extremely fearful of leaving home, was increasingly ritualistic in his daily routines (which travel threatened), and had become very mistrustful of strangers and suspected that they might have "unseemly motives." With treatment of his depression he felt much better and within three months they booked a cruise to Alaska, which was a pleasure for both of them. And true to her word, Mrs. I felt "fit as a fiddle" the whole trip!

Another type of loss for aging couples is loss of friends and family. Indeed, fortitude about the inevitability of death as people age only partly soothes the pain of yet another death of a sibling or childhood friend. As one seventy-three-year-old physician patient of mine (who had just returned from his fifty-year medical school reunion) said: "There's only a few of us left now. If I live long enough, I don't know if I've got the heart to attend my sixtieth—too much sadness, too much to have to accept over one weekend."

In the previous section I noted the loss of one's professional identity and the challenge for physicians to come to terms with this—a tall order for individuals like Dr. P, whose self-esteem was largely dictated by his status and accomplishments as an academic physician. For male physicians, retiring is not only the loss of one's role in society but also the loss of one's gender role as a man, as a worker, as a breadwinner, as the head of one's family. There is a corresponding shift to more tenuous or informal roles in the family, but this takes time and may be only moderately successful for some physicians.

Lidz,[2] writing in a metaphorical vein, described old age as autumn, not winter: a time of contentment, and a time to gather the harvest.

Contrasting aging with adolescence, there is a waning of one's sexual drive and functioning. We turn to the past as opposed to looking forward; we reflect upon what we've accomplished and experienced. There is increased dependency on one's children and others of the succeeding generation. And unlike adolescents, who are moving toward intimacy with someone else, aging men and women must sooner or later absorb the loss of the person with whom they have shared their lives.

This psychological process, or something akin to it, may form the substrate of marital symptoms that break out in aging physician couples. On the surface are complaints such as frequent arguments or bickering, poor communication, overdrinking in one or both, lack of affection, and distancing. Underneath, however, they are struggling with many challenges of "autumn." Examples that come to mind are (a) when one of the individuals has a terminal illness and is dying—instead of gaining closeness and mutual support through this time period, they fight a lot and avoid each other to cover the painful and imminent reality of losing each other; (b) when one of the partners is more contemplative and insightful than the other—he or she wants to talk about the melancholy of their losses and the other won't listen because it is too frightening; and (c) when one of the partners is much older than the other—the former is at a life stage that is punctuated by loss, but the latter is not and cannot understand, leading to a pungent loneliness and sadness about their marriage.

COMPETENCY TO PRACTICE MEDICINE

Aging as a physician is a bit of a paradox. While one's breadth of experience as a clinician expands and enhances diagnostic and therapeutic expertise, there is a simultaneous constriction of one's endurance for long hours and middle-of-the-night awakenings, memory, and technical ability. Some physicians are very aware of this, acknowledge it, and take steps to avoid mishaps and accidents. Unfortunately, not all physicians know when they are not practicing medicine safely or carefully. Further, they may be completely oblivious or unresponsive to overtures by well-meaning office assistants, nurses, physician colleagues, and family members that they are concerned about their competency. Nothing is done then until there is a formal complaint from a patient, a patterns of practice committee, or a hospital audit committee— or a lawsuit charging malpractice.

Incompetency to practice is on a continuum from mild to severe. The physician may be simply out of date and not practicing modern medicine—he or she has not kept up through continuing medical education (reading, hospital rounds, courses, updates, and so forth) and uses diagnostic tests, medications, and treatment strategies that have been supplanted by newer and better ones. The physician may be burned out and is frequently out of sorts, forgetful, late, irritable, seemingly uncaring, and overextended. Patients and coworkers complain about his or her behavior. The physician may show a pattern of increasingly frequent "near misses": errors in dosages on prescriptions and hospital orders, bleeding problems in the operating room, complications from anesthetics during recovery, attrition in patients who do not feel comfortable with the care rendered, or an ever-lengthening file of patient complaints to the licensing body or department chair. Or the physician is found to be completely dangerous because of personal illness (e.g., Alzheimer's disease and other kinds of dementia, alcohol intoxication, toxic brain syndromes of various causes, or mania).

What has this got to do with marriage? A lot! Usually spouses are worried sick and have felt powerless to influence their husband or wife to stop practicing medicine before someone is harmed or killed. Some will call the "physician well-being" hotline that is available in all states and provinces. But many do not know where to turn, especially if they lead a rather isolated marriage in a small medical community. There is also a pronounced, and alarming, tendency for family members of disabled doctors to deny and rationalize, thereby enabling the continuation of incompetent patterns (so-called codependency).

Marital problems may be either a contributing factor in charges of incompetency to practice medicine or a consequence. I will discuss ways in which marital disharmony contributes first. If a physician is aging but also has an ongoing unhappy marriage, there may be a tendency for the physician to overwork instead of dealing with marital troubles head-on. There may not be enough leisure in the physician's life as more and more of his or her identity is wrapped up in being a physician. This is a risk factor for medical mishaps. Further, if physicians' marriages are not good, they may not be able to rely on their spouses to "monitor" their practices and their professional activities. They may be leading separate lives, and their spouses wouldn't even notice if they were working night and day, or never reading medical journals, or drinking too much, or even developing symptoms of a brain disorder. Without this kind of reality check or consensual validation, physicians who are incompetent or becoming so may go unnoticed for months, especially in solo practice situations.

Another way in which marital troubles can contribute to incompetency to practice is through illness. More specifically, marital discord, especially if it is severe and unrelenting, can make people sick. Hence, if the physician who is aging already has some biological factors playing a role in his or her judgment, cognitive integrity, and memory, then marital discord may accentuate the underlying difficulty. This may lead to severe depression, drug taking, alcohol overuse, insomnia, and so forth—all of which may cause the physician to make medical mistakes.

But what about incompetency allegations or charges that cause marital discord? In this situation there is a perceived or real threat to one's license to practice medicine and hence one's professional livelihood. This can have severe financial implications, especially if there is no good financial planning, no other income, and heavy indebtedness. If the physician is not allowed to practice medicine or can do so only in a reduced capacity, this calls for a high level of understanding and adjustment on the spouse's part. Worry, anger, and misunderstanding may cause marital spats and withdrawing.

Another type of marital problem is rooted in humiliation and dishonor. When physicians are charged with incompetence, either through licensing bodies or the courts, and this information becomes public, there is always shame. For physicians and their families to live with this may be exceedingly difficult. Even the most solid of marriages may be severely tested, and compromised, through the long period of licensure investigation and final deliberation.

A third type of marital discord stemming from competency to practice matters is related to loss, as I discussed earlier. What I am referring to is aggregate loss that becomes overwhelming and causes marital unhappiness. If the physician is ill, acutely or chronically and perhaps irreversibly (e.g., Alzheimer's disease), then there is loss of his or her good health, not just competence to practice medicine and earn a living. And if the physician is becoming demented and there are marital troubles, even the chances of marital therapy being effective are greatly reduced, except in the early stages of the illness. What is more helpful then is for the physician's spouse to receive supportive psychotherapy addressed to living with someone with a disabling, and terminal, neuropsychiatric disorder.

In the early stages of Alzheimer's disease, the changes may be so subtle or masked that the diagnosis may be missed. Here is an example:

When Mrs. F and her husband, Dr. F, came for their initial visit, these were her words: "He's impossible to live with, and unless something changes, I'm moving in with my sister. We've been to two marriage counselors already and things aren't any better." Mrs. F explained that her husband had changed over the previous two years from "my best friend" into "a complete stranger."

She complained that he had become selfish and thoughtless toward her (no wedding anniversary card, no acknowledgment of an award she had won for her volunteerism), that he yelled at her one minute and was silent and withdrawn the next, that he had become "lazy" about his clothes and grooming (he wouldn't shine his shoes anymore and some days he didn't shave before going to the office), that he picked fights with her and used language that was crude and out of character for him, and that he had become totally obsessed with winning the lottery, spending a lot of money each week on several tickets (which Mrs. F would find in the car, in Dr. F's suits, in his black medical bag, and a couple of times stuffed in with his tennis gear).

In response to his wife's concerns, Dr. F merely stated: "I don't need to explain a thing. If Marie doesn't want to live with me anymore, so be it. I can manage fine on my own." He said these words without any emotional expression. Mrs. F began to cry and angrily stated, "Yes, when you can't even boil water, or run the washing machine, you're going to manage just fine." Dr. F rejoined, "You see, doctor, this is what I live with—sarcasm and put-downs." The remainder of my visit with the two of them was more of this, so I arranged individual visits with each of them for the following day to do a more thorough assessment.

Both Dr. and Mrs. F were sixty-four years old. They had been married for thirty-eight years and had four grown children. There had been no marital troubles of any significance until recently. My examination of Dr. F, corroborated by his son (a radiologist) and his office staff (who were very concerned about his work performance and who had complained to no avail to his associate in the office), was strongly suggestive of early dementia. I referred him to a neurologist for investigation of this, and Alzheimer's disease was confirmed. The rest of my therapeutic work with Dr. and Mrs. F was largely supportive and explanatory, although he needed to take an antidepressant a few months later, in part related to his despondency about having to give up practicing medicine.

REMARRIAGE IN OLDER PHYSICIANS

In Chapter Five I discussed common dynamics for men who divorce in midlife and remarry someone much younger. In this section, I want to describe remarriage problems in older physicians, both men and women, who are divorced or widowed. Before I discuss problems, let me emphasize that most remarriages in the later years of life are happy and fulfilling ones for both parties.

Some couples who divorce in their later years have been miserable together for as long as they can remember.[3] Unlike many of their peers whose marriages improved once the children grew up and left home, their marriages remained static or worsened as the years passed. Efforts to stay together by sheer will, determination, or habit have not succeeded, and divorce becomes inevitable. The person who initiates and wants the separation usually feels guilty and responsible for the other's welfare. This means that he or she will want to ensure that there is plenty of support—both financially and psychologically—for the spouse.

Also, older individuals who want to leave their marriages frequently are of very different temperament than their spouses. They may be quite optimistic and forward-looking in disposition and keen to approach their remaining years with gusto, rather than resignation. They usually also enjoy good health. Often their spouses are not like this but are more passive, conservative, and cautious. Here is an example:[4]

Dr. W was referred to me by his family physician, who was worried about his mental state, in particular his judgment. He wondered if Dr. W might be "hypomanic or going senile" because of his persistent desire to leave his marriage. Dr. W was an eighty-two-year-old retired dentist and university professor who had been married for fifty-nine years and who had five children, all married and out of the home. I conducted a careful and thorough assessment of Dr. W over a series of appointments that included a detailed personal and family history, marital history, medical evaluation, and mental status examination, especially of his cognitive and affective functioning. Dr. W was in superb physical and mental health—but he was indeed unhappily married and had been so for a long time. I had only to listen to him with an open mind (and an open heart, I might add) as he gently described his subjective sense of sadness, loneliness, and restlessness to begin to appreciate his dilemma. His words were poignant: "It's terrible to be thought of as having a screw loose because you want to leave your marriage at eighty-two years of age. If I were forty years younger, no one would bat an eye. I admit I'm being selfish, but I have only a few years left on this earth, and I still have a lot to accomplish. I can't do these things if I remain married." Dr. W did separate, and this was eased by my working not only with him but also with his wife and his children for several months.

I interviewed Mrs. W shortly after Dr. W told her that he was leaving but before he actually moved out. Her husband's decision to leave did not come as a complete surprise, since he had spoken about separation at many points over the years. She too was unhappily married and had many complaints about her husband but never seriously considered leaving herself. At one level she was relieved, since she had felt "on hold" for a long time. But she also admitted that she was nervous about being on her own (she was fearful of intruders in her neighborhood and fearful that if she became sick, no one would be im-

mediately available to help). A private woman, Mrs. W had many concerns about what to tell her friends and what her neighbors might think about her husband's departure.

Dr. W adjusted quickly to the separation. He began traveling a lot, became more active at his community center, enrolled in a creative writing course, and did volunteer work. I only saw him a couple of visits. On the other hand, I saw Mrs. W for several months. She attended a psychiatric day program for a couple of months, and that was helpful for her. It alleviated her sense of rejection and isolation. On two occasions, I met with her two daughters. They were very angry at their father. I think it helped them just to ventilate about the loss of family.

Dr. W did not remarry. Here is another example of an older and widowed physician who did:

Dr. E did not come for marital therapy but for treatment of depression. Her unhappy and unfulfilling marriage was the major contributor to her feelings of despondency, guilt, sleeplessness, weight loss, and lack of energy. What she had difficulty doing was admitting this to herself.

Dr. E had been married for only two years. She was seventy years old and a retired cardiologist. Her first husband had died ten years earlier in a plane crash. Losing him was devastating for her—they were great companions, had lots of common interests, deeply loved their six grandchildren, and had plans to travel extensively when they both retired. Unfortunately, his tragic death occurred first. By the time that Dr. E met Dr. G (six years after her husband's death), she was longing for a committed relationship and someone with whom to share her many interests.

Dr. G was a retired dentist, and he was the same age as Dr. E. Unfortunately, within weeks of their wedding, Dr. G had a heart attack—and he never fully recovered. Despite clearance from his personal cardiologist that he had healed nicely, Dr. G continued to have chest pains, periods of shortness of breath, feelings of panic, and fearfulness of venturing much beyond his home and neighborhood. Dr. E concluded that her husband might be depressed, but he refused to consider this or go to see a psychiatrist. Over the next couple of years he became more of a recluse, and Dr. E became more angry, resentful, and depressed. All of her hopes and dreams to have a companion had vanished.

Dr. E began to feel better relatively quickly with psychotherapy, once she realized that she had some choice in her health. She began to consider separation as an option, and this is what she eventually did (she had hoped that her husband would at least try marital therapy with her, but he refused this as well). She did not feel "like a failure" as much as she feared she would. Within months she was leading a very full life as a woman on her own.

When aging physicians remarry, this can be an upsetting time for their adult children, as well as the adult children of the new partner. What are some of the issues? First, it helps tremendously if the children like and respect the person whom their mother or father is marrying, which is not always the case. Sometimes this is because the parties really don't know each other very well so that their relationship is largely impressionistic, third-hand, or superficial. Sometimes the adult children's concern about their parents' judgment is well taken, however, in that the two individuals are not well matched and there are many areas of actual or potential incompatibility. Understandably, given the nature of adult children's roles with their parents, they feel somewhat protective and may behave in quite a controlling manner, which may alienate the parents.

Second, something more self-serving and sinister occurs when adult children exploit their aging parent(s) financially. They may view any person that their mother or father intends to marry with suspicion and as an interloper. They are usually concerned about losing out on any perquisites that they are receiving (financial support, use of the family cottage, babysitting, etc.) or anticipate receiving by inheritance. Their worst fear is that they will be cut off completely and not receive a cent.

Third, some adult children have not come to terms with the loss of the other parent, if that parent has died. This is especially so if their mother or father has not been dead very long. If the remaining parent is quite serious about someone new, and plans to marry, all of this may be too quick or seem inappropriate for the son or daughter. In their personal grieving, they cannot appreciate the loneliness of their mother or father, and their strong need to be recoupled. Widowers tend to remarry sooner than widows; so when fathers remarry, this situation may sorely test the maturity, patience, flexibility, and good humor of their children.

Fourth, when aging divorced physicians remarry, this may be hard for one or all of the children, who feel a conflict of loyalty with their other parent. In other words, if their mother or father has not moved on or resolved many of the unpleasant feelings associated with divorce, it may be extremely difficult for the children to welcome the other parent's new partner or spouse. They feel in some ways that they are betraying their mother or father, and this may make them feel guilty. This matter may become even more complicated when adult children have their own unresolved anger or hurt with the parent who is now coupled. They are not likely then to give the new individual in their mom or dad's life a fair chance and may even refuse to attend the wedding or acknowledge the union in any way.

CONCLUSION

I have attempted to outline some of the challenges of aging that older physicians must confront, and how these challenges may affect their marriages. Marital problems that arise in one's later years are not uncommon, and it is important that mental health professionals be aware of this. For too long there has been a blindness to the psychological and social factors that aggravate the health problems of aging physicians, and many of their marriages have been unexamined and untreated. It is time now to do something about that.

REFERENCES

1. Ellen M. Berman and Harold I. Lief, "Marital Therapy from a Psychiatric Perspective: An Overview," *American Journal of Psychiatry* 132 (1975), 583–592.
2. Theodore Lidz, "Phases of Adult Life: An Overview," in *Mid-Life: Developmental and Clinical Issues,* ed. W. H. Norman and T. J. Scaramella (New York: Brunner/Mazel, 1980), 20–37.
3. Michael F. Myers, *Men and Divorce* (New York: Guilford, 1989).
4. Ibid., 90–91.

Chapter Seven

SPECIAL PROBLEMS

In this chapter, I want to discuss some of the special problems that can occur in the lives of doctors and their spouses. The focus here will be on those problems that, for the most part, are external to the marriage yet are so upsetting that they do affect marital functioning and happiness. Further, these are problems that are not predictable; they can happen to anyone. They may beset couples with no intrinsic marital discord or couples who are already on shaky ground before the added stress occurs. Needless to say, the couple's ability to cope with special problems is predicated upon the resting state of their marriage before the change, their prior experience in dealing with adversity, and the magnitude of the stress.

MEDICAL ILLNESS IN THE DOCTOR, SPOUSE, OR CHILD

When Dr. M first consulted me she was forty years old and had been suffering from rheumatoid arthritis for ten years. Her affliction was severe and relentless, for despite careful attention to her rheumatologist's prescribed drug regimen and life-style changes, Dr. M was not doing all that well. By the end of her working day as a family physician she was quite exhausted and complained that she felt "a hundred years old." Dr. M had gradually reduced the hours of practice because of this fatigue as well as severe joint stiffness and reduced mobility in the mornings. She had to give up obstetrics, minor surgical procedures, and other tasks that required good manual dexterity. Despite this, though, she continued to enjoy practicing medicine, found it fulfilling, and liked the other doctors with whom she was associated in her office.

Dr. M's main worry was her marriage. Although she and her husband, an accountant, had no obvious difficulties, she remained concerned. In fact, it was precisely this that worried her—they never argued, they never fought, but they also were doing less and less as a couple. This alarmed her not only because they used to do a lot together (they had no children, by choice) but also because she felt largely responsible for this change. Because of her increasing physical discomfort and her fatigue, she stopped going to chamber music concerts, plays, and other events that they used to share and enjoy together. Her husband never complained about going alone. Nor did he complain about their increasingly insular social world; at one time they entertained a lot, but now they rarely had friends in or accepted invitations to attend parties and functions. Two years earlier she had given up bridge, one of her favorite pastimes.

Another worry for Dr. M was the deterioration in their sexual relationship with each other. She could not remember when they last made love. Again, she blamed herself. She admitted that she had absolutely no physical desire for sex but that she felt "psychologically interested." What she meant by this was that she loved her husband, found him physically appealing, and most of the time thought she would feel receptive to his overtures. She herself had lost all assertiveness for initiating sex; some of this loss was because of fatigue and the fact that she was living with pain. Most critically, much of this sexual reluctance was secondary to her altered body image. She felt terrible about her body, no longer felt attractive or sexy, and feared ultimate rejection by her husband.

Dr. M did well with only a few supportive psychotherapy visits, and her mood and outlook picked up. I also saw her and her husband together for a brief course of marital therapy. Each of them had been sitting on a lot of feelings, especially loss, disappointment, and anger. Their communication improved, and so did their sexual relationship.

What this example illustrates is twofold: (1) Chronic debilitating illness affects the individual emotionally and behaviorally, and (2) it also affects the individual's partner. Living with someone who is ill is always difficult to a lesser or greater degree. There is usually a mixture of feelings—sadness and concern for one's partner, closely aligned with more unpleasant feelings such as despondency and resentment that this is even happening. "Why you?" and "Why me?" are part of the picture. Mr. W, Dr. M's husband, felt a lot of resentment and self-pity deep inside, but he never shared these feelings with his wife. In typical fashion, he did not want to "hurt her more than she was hurting already." What he didn't realize was that his withdrawal—of interest, affection, and sexual desire—was hurting her just as much, if not more.

Quite understandably, individuals with a chronic disorder that is progressively worsening can become preoccupied with it and turn inward. This morbid egocentricity is based in part on the large number of symptoms the person has, in part on the time-consuming treatment(s), and in part on the demoralization that accompanies the illness. What happens is that the individual does not and/or cannot give much to his or her spouse. Mr. W felt that Dr. M had become very self-absorbed and rarely asked about him or expressed interest in him. He felt rejected sexually by her; he felt that she saw him as just another bother, another obstacle in her life. Because he didn't want to hurt her, he didn't say anything about these feelings. When he was permitted to express his feelings in a conjoint session with Dr. M, he felt less burdened, and she felt better informed about his quietly hostile and aloof manner toward her.

Male physicians handle illness in a way that may be characteristic of both their sex and their profession.

Dr. F, a forty-year-old radiologist, came to see me, albeit reluctantly, six months after a severe coronary. He started the visit by saying, "I'm fine. It's my wife who needs to be here. She says I'm driving her nuts." Since his coronary, Dr. F had become totally preoccupied with his health and his recovery. He had lost thirty pounds of excess weight, and he read constantly about cardiovascular disease. The diet he now consumed was extremely rigid and very restrictive in salt, carbohydrates, and cholesterol. Efforts of his cardiologist and nutritionist to get him to relax a bit on this diet were unsuccessful. Meals at home had become a power struggle; his wife could no longer prepare anything that he found acceptable. Most of the time he cross-examined her about the ingredients. She blew up at him frequently; he began making his own meals and eating apart from his wife and children.

Behind Dr. F's obsessional behavior was tremendous anxiety, which he was slowly able to talk about after a few low-key and nonthreatening visits with me. He felt marked—and scarred—for the rest of his life. He no longer felt "normal" or part of the mainstream. Further, his attempts to talk about his feelings with his wife and his friends were not well received; he felt that their statements of reassurance and understanding were manifestations of their own anxiety and inability to listen to him. Consequently, he felt more and more isolated and misunderstood. He lived in constant fear of another coronary and certain death.

I diagnosed Dr. F as having an anxiety disorder. Despite a lot of moodiness, he was not clinically depressed.

I do not want to overgeneralize, but this example illustrates how many male doctors react to threat, that is, in a rigid, obsessional, and controlling manner. These reactions have repercussions for the marriage because it is very hard to live with this kind of behavior. When I saw Dr. F and his wife together, it became very clear that each felt unheard, unappreciated, and angry at the other. Dr. F's wife had her own anxiety about losing him, which she wanted to discuss with him, but she felt shut out. Once they were able to appreciate how their ways of coping with this life-threatening stress were bouncing off one another,

and they could begin to relax again, their ability to communicate returned to normal.

What about medical illness in the spouses of doctors? In what ways
can sickness affect these marriages? I'll begin with the situation in which
it is the doctor's wife with a medical disorder. As a psychiatrist subspecialized in marital therapy, I find that I am most likely to hear about
the impact of medical illness some time after the fact, down the road a
few months or years when the couple comes for treatment. Classically,
the doctor's wife has never felt that her husband cares about or has
much sympathy for her when she is medically ill. Examples include not
listening to her symptoms or dismissing them as "nothing to worry
about"; calling her neurotic or hypochondriacal; not asking her about
her visit(s) to her doctor; not taking time off work when she is home
sick; not visiting her much when she is in the hospital—or visiting only
during the day while he is there making rounds; not being attentive or
available during her pregnancies, labor, deliveries, and postpartum days
(this is rare now, but was not unusual before the 1970s).

Being ignored when she is medically ill is one aspect of a larger
problem for some doctors' wives; these women may be ignored much of
the time in their marriages. I talked about this in Chapter Two. In such
marriages, these women are expected to be strong and understanding at
all times. Medicine is their husbands' first priority, and they are supposed to understand that. Usually the marriages are traditional in form:
The man's work, and its attendant status and financial return, and
compelling nature, is all important; the woman's work in the home,
although deemed important, is unpaid and of lesser status.

*Dr. B pulled me aside one day in the hospital corridor and asked me if
I could see his wife. He had just learned the day before that she was abusing
tranquilizers (benzodiazepines) and had been for several months. His hope was
that with my assistance she could "stop being so silly." I noted that he was not
only worried about her but annoyed at himself, saying, "How could I have
missed it?" I agreed to see her within a day or two but made it clear that
I might eventually need to work with both of them if there were underlying marital issues. He replied that he would be quite willing to come in with
her if necessary.*

*Mrs. B did very well with individual treatment and was off tranquilizers
within six weeks by a gradual and careful reduction of her daily dosages of
medication. She was relieved and felt better about herself. She was now in touch
with a lot of angry feelings toward her husband. She was especially angry
about his inability to appreciate her situation and his lack of interest in trying
to explore with her possible reasons for her anxiety and unhappiness, which led*

to the drug taking in the first place. He tended instead to do two things that really bothered her: He watched her closely for signs of drug usage, occasionally "grilling" her, and he responded judgmentally whenever their talks together referred back to the period of self-medicating.

When I saw Dr. B alone I was able to get a clearer understanding of his feelings about his wife's use of drugs. He really was dumbfounded, and it made absolutely no sense to him. He saw his wife as very capable and very strong. "That's why I married her, because I knew she would have a very important and responsible job running the house, raising the children, maintaining her appearance, and entertaining with style" were his words. His rejoinder to my question about her possible isolation in the home and loneliness in the marriage (he worked long hours and traveled a lot to meetings) was, "No, that's not like her to become stressed." I came to realize that this man, for the moment, had a lot of difficulty accepting human vulnerability in his wife; he was still denying a great deal and was disappointed and angry at her for not being "perfect." For her to feel anxious or down was totally unacceptable to him.

There may be many reasons why a physician is unsympathetic to his wife's health problems. First, his reaction may be typical of his manner toward medical illness in his patients—cool, objective, clinical, and professional. Second, he may be a perfectionist in his outlook; he does not accept illness in himself or in his family. Third, as a doctor his professional socialization has been to always put medicine first before his wife and children; he does not have the time and energy to give to their health care needs. And fourth, his wife may not be direct and forthright in admitting and explaining her illness, pain, and so forth. This reluctance may be a manifestation of her personality, that is, she may hate to bother others, needs to be self-reliant, or feels unworthy.

Let me turn now to the situation in which doctors' husbands are medically ill. I want to make two points. The first has to do with women as caretakers and is a concern when the woman physician treats her own husband and does not insist that he seek independent medical care. This is linked sometimes with my second observation, which is that many doctors' husbands refuse to see a physician (like men in general). What happens next is that the woman physician gets seduced into diagnosing and treating her husband because she is so worried about him. The commonest situation is providing her husband with various kinds of medication, including tranquilizers, painkillers, and sleeping pills.

When the doctor's child is ill some of these dynamics come into play; they can cause misunderstandings and tension in marriages. Some doctors regularly and inappropriately (in my mind) treat their own children. At one time, when doctors were scarce or separated by geographical distance, this was necessary to relieve suffering and perhaps to save a child's life; it constituted good medical judgment. Nowadays, except in rural and isolated areas, other physicians are never very far away. Typically, it is the doctor's wife who takes the child to the doctor's office, or clinic, or hospital. Her husband may actually be poorly informed about the symptoms, diagnosis, and medical management because he has not been present at the child's visit(s) to the doctor. Either the father assumes he knows what is going on because he is a doctor himself, or it is assumed by his wife and the child's doctor that he knows. If his child is hospitalized, he may visit only during his "working day." These visits may actually be convenient and give him more time with his son or daughter, but because he is in a work mode, he may not really be there emotionally. Further, he talks to the treating doctor more as a colleague and fellow professional rather than as the worried father of a sick child.

Some doctors' wives come to resent bearing complete and total responsibility for attending to their children's health. This is especially so when, or if, the child has a chronic and debilitating illness that involves many visits to various specialists, special needs in the school, and extra time and one-to-one work in the home, as in cases of cystic fibrosis, rheumatoid arthritis, heart disease, and various neurological disorders. These women need the moral support of their physician husbands; they need to be given a break from time to time; and they need their husbands' actual physical assistance with driving, meetings, and treatments. There is a risk of fragmentation in these families—because of the time-intensive nature of the illness, the mother and child become tightly bound emotionally, and the physician father is off on the sidelines. Both the man and his son or daughter lose because they do not have the emotional connectedness that comes with the many hours of daily contact around the illness.

"PROBLEM CHILD"

I am using the term *problem child* loosely here to refer to any child of a physician with a long-standing or recurrent problem that is a cause of worry. This worry may be for the child's safety, physical health, mental health, academic functioning, and future as a happy and self-supporting adult. There are many of these, and I will list a few: any of the physically disabling illnesses mentioned earlier; attention deficit disorders, for instance, the various learning disabilities with or without hyperactivity; mental retardation; cerebral palsy; eating disorders; alcohol and drug abuse; bipolar affective disorder; schizophrenia; and various disorders of conduct and behavior, such as stealing, truancy, and fighting. These problems must not be underestimated in their ability to wreak havoc on a family and totally destroy its happiness, integrity, and purpose.

Dr. and Mrs. T were referred to me for marital therapy by their son Adam's psychiatrist. Dr. G was treating Adam for severe hyperactivity, learning difficulties, and aggressive behavior both at home and at school. Dr. G was concerned about the parents' increasing difficulty in coping with Adam. She found them less responsive to her instructions regarding medication and to her attempts at counseling. She admitted that Adam was one of her more difficult patients and certainly a handful for any family, but she wondered if the parents' marital difficulties were both contributing to as well as a result of Adam's problems. She was right!

Dr. T had a lot of difficulty accepting Adam's diagnosis despite his knowledge of attention deficit disorder and his respect for Dr. G. He admitted that he was very disappointed and angry at having a son with a problem. He realized this made him irritable and impatient with Adam; he yelled frequently, was verbally abusive, and punished his son physically. He always felt apologetic and guilty later. He tried to come to terms with this anger by decreasing his time with Adam. He worked harder in his medical practice and took on committee and community work. Mrs. T was much more in touch with Adam's limitations, and for the most part she handled him well. However, she too got weary and was bitter that her husband was "copping out" and leaving so much to her. Her resentment had become generalized by the time I met with the two of them. To make matters worse, in their individual sessions with me, both confessed to being emotionally and sexually involved with another person outside their marriage. Neither had told the other, nor did either suspect the other.

Let me give another example:

When I saw Dr. and Dr. N, they had been married for thirty-five years. Their chief complaint was, "We've come to see if there's any hope for us." What they described was a fluctuating pattern of marital tension, fighting, and unhappiness for the fifteen years since their son Paul was diagnosed as having schizophrenia (later changed to manic–depressive illness) at the age of eighteen. And what a time they had had with him! He had been hospitalized involuntarily on many occasions, had lived off and on at home and halfway houses, and was poorly responsive to drug treatment. He had never been able to complete college or hold down a job. He was also violent and threatened both of them when psychotic. Many psychiatrists of different theoretical and therapeutic schools had been consulted over the years. Dr. and Dr. N had received lots of different kinds of advice and counseling, including implicit and explicit statements that they were to blame for his illness. It was only in the previous five years that their son was being treated by a very sensible, and sensitive, psychiatrist who appreciated the intrinsic nature of Paul's illness and who was available, supportive, and kind to these confused and distraught parents. In fact, it was this psychiatrist who suggested marital therapy for them.

Dr. and Dr. N did very well with a combination of conjoint and individual visits. They were able to stop scapegoating the marriage for all their anxieties about Paul's disease. This change included letting go of self-blame and blaming the other. Both needed to mourn their hopes and longings for Paul; they slowly came to accept his very severe disability. They had to step aside a bit, become a bit more selfish, and look at their personal and interpersonal needs in the marriage. Indeed, they began to do more together as a couple; for the first time in years they were able to truly smile and laugh. They rekindled a love that had lain dormant for a very long time.

Anorexia nervosa is an eating disorder that is more common in upper-middle-class and high-achieving families. It is therefore not uncommon in adolescent daughters of physicians and, more recently, in women medical students.[1] Depending upon its severity (anorexia nervosa has a significant mortality rate of 5%–21.5%),[2] having a daughter with the disease can be quite a worry and lead to marital misunderstandings and conflict. Anorexia nervosa can also be exacerbated by parental distress, separation, and divorce. What is becoming increasingly evident is that family behavior is as much a response to the illness as a contributing factor in causation.[3]

Amy was sixteen years old and slightly overweight when she began dieting to get down to what she considered a normal weight for her. However, like so many teenage girls with anorexia nervosa, she didn't stop at her desired weight but kept going. She stopped menstruating when her weight dipped below ninety pounds on her 5'1" frame. She enjoyed being thin and "the envy of all my friends." More importantly, she enjoyed being in control and the feeling of mastery and power she had over her eating. Before this began, she considered herself powerless, not just with food, but with everything in her life.

Amy's father was an internist, her mother a teacher. When they came to see me, they were on the verge of separating but did not want to proceed without assistance. They felt that their marital difficulties antedated Amy's eating disorder by many years. They both were very knowledgeable about anorexia nervosa; both had read a lot about it and had looked inward at their personal and marital conflicts and the possible role of this conflict in eating disorders. They felt that their remaining together was making Amy's condition worse. They also felt that they would react to her defiance and deception around food much more calmly if they weren't bouncing off each other. I had to agree, albeit tentatively, because on all their visits to my office they were so tense, always sparring with each other. They reported that they were like this "all the time now."

Amy's parents did separate and eventually divorced. Although she was hospitalized once during the first year of separation, she responded well to medication, behavior therapy, and family therapy. As the separation became more obviously permanent, she became progressively better. She maintained a weight on the thin side of normal, her periods returned, and she became more self-assured about her appearance and her relationships with others. She felt better and happier. So did each of her parents.

DEATH OF A CHILD

The death of a child is always a devastating tragedy for a family and has profound effects on the parents as individuals and on their marriage. Parents feel grief for a long period of time, they think about their child, and they may have issues involving the child that were not resolved before his or her death. They search for reasons for their child's death for months, maybe years. Most look for meaning in life and death and grow in many areas of their lives.[4] Many grow closer to their immediate and extended families.[5]

There are, however, a significant number of couples who do not do well. These couples become severely symptomatic, tension erupts, and they separate—some temporarily, some permanently—anywhere from one to five years after their child's death. Some, but not all, couples are already having difficulties before their child's death; the trauma is so severe that their relationship cannot withstand it.

I have seen several distressed medical couples in my practice who have lost a child at some point in their marriage. Sometimes their chief complaint is that they cannot come to terms with their child's death. The loss is usually more recent for these couples. Other couples give the death of their child (or antecedent illness, if their child did not die suddenly) as a reference point for their marital difficulty—that is, their lives together changed markedly then and have not been the same since. Still other couples describe the loss of their child as just one of many losses in their lives together. They do not wish to minimize its sting, but to place this loss in perspective with regard to their present ill health.

For example, I once saw a doctor and his wife who in the previous five years had these losses: his mother died, her brother died, they moved away from their family and friends for fellowship training, he failed his specialty boards, they had a miscarriage at two months, then a stillborn child, and now were separated!

One of the most common complaints of couples who have had a child die is a breakdown in their communication with each other. In the early weeks and months of bereavement this breakdown is quite common and normal; each of them is grieving privately with or without the assistance of family, friends, or counselors. However, when they are completely unable to talk with each other about their child and to share their "grief work," alienation and separateness may become serious. This alienation may then extend to other areas of their lives together so that they hardly communicate on any level or do anything together. Individually, each is feeling many painful emotions—shock, numbness, rage, sorrow, and guilt among them.

Dr. and Mrs. E had been married for twenty-four years when their eighteen-year-old son, Sean, was killed in a boating accident. Two years later I was asked to see Mrs. E for depression. She was very ill. She had become a complete recluse, spending most of her day in her room; she had lost twenty pounds, her sleep was disturbed, and she longed for death. Previously a virtual teetotaler, she was now abusing alcohol. She required hospitalization and electroconvulsive therapy, to which she responded well. Maintenance antidepressant medication and supportive psychotherapy enabled her to resume many of her usual activities and to find new purpose in living.

At this point, both Mrs. E and Dr. E, in separate visits, were able to talk about Sean's death and how losing him had affected each of them and their relationship. One of the reasons why they were unable to really discuss his death together in any depth or to comfort one another was because of the anger and blame they felt toward each other. Understandably, both felt terribly guilty about these feelings, so they said nothing. Mrs. E resented Dr. E for throwing himself into his work immediately after Sean's death "as if nothing had happened, as if Sean never existed." She went on to say, "I know he's hurting inside, I know this is his way of coping, and I know a lot of doctors cope with personal tragedy this way, but I hate it and I hate him for it." Dr. E had a lot of anger toward his wife—he resented her "for feeling sorry for herself; for letting Sean down by caving in; and for becoming a drunk." What was more remarkable about my work with these two was that after they were able to discharge much of their pent-up anger and guilt in their individual visits with me, they were able to reconnect with an intensity and mutual joy that was extremely moving. Dr. E summed it up this way: "I feel we've been adrift in our own lifeboats for two and a half years—adrift in a foggy sea—I never thought we'd see each other again." I do not know if he was conscious of his use of a marine metaphor and its symbolic attachment to Sean's death by drowning.

Let me give another example of the impact of a child's death on a medical couple:

Don and Diane were both family physicians who were already in marital therapy with me and about to separate when their second child, Molly, age four months, died of sudden infant death syndrome (SIDS). This terrible loss, with its massive guilt for both of them, was overwhelming. They managed to remain together for almost nine months after their daughter's death, partly to try to avoid another upset for their four-year-old son and partly to avoid the antici-pated disapproval of their respective families. But they could no longer bear remaining together. Their separation was not only inevitable but lifesaving. The complicating factor for Don and Diane was that nobody knew how troubled and barren their marriage was before their daughter died. In fact, they were close to separating when Diane suddenly found herself pregnant with Molly. They decided to remain together and things improved, but only for a few months. Don met another woman toward the end of Diane's pregnancy and remained involved with her for several months. This woman broke up with him just before Molly's death. As one can see, this couple was experiencing tremendous behind-the-scenes stress that greatly complicated their lives. They already felt like failures in their marriage and now they began to struggle with feelings of failure as parents. Fortunately, each remained in individual therapy with me for a while after they separated. They have a joint custody arrangement for their son and have created and maintained one of the most successful and mutu-ally respectful co-parenting relationships that I've experienced in my profes-sional career.

GAY SON OR LESBIAN DAUGHTER

Learning about and coming to terms with their son's gayness or daughter's lesbianism is another type of special problem for physicians and their spouses that I want to discuss. Regardless of their degree of preparedness for the disclosure, most parents find the news that their son is gay or their daughter lesbian jarring. Often the parents them-selves have reactions that vary in intensity and duration. One parent may adjust and adapt quickly, while the other has a very difficult time.

Dr. and Mrs. A came in together. Two years previously, their twenty-three-year-old son had told his father he was gay. The father, with the son's encouragement, told the mother. Although two years had passed, Mrs. A stated that she still had trouble accepting her son's style of living. Her reaction had caused estrangement and a great deal of secretive behavior on the son's part. Mrs. A disapproved of most of her son's friends and refused to meet them if he brought them by the family home. (He had been living on his own for three years.) During the interview, Mrs. A confided, with her husband's coaxing, that she felt responsible for the son's sexual orientation and could not help but feel it was all her fault. Dr. A, who stated that he felt more accepting than his wife, explained that his acceptance was the result of having met and treated gay people in his practice. Mrs. A admitted she had had no exposure to homosexuals whatsoever. She said she felt as if she were living in the Dark Ages.[6]

Mrs. A, like many parents of gay and lesbian children, felt guilty and blamed herself. This emotion is often closely aligned with anger, or is camouflaged or overshadowed by anger. I mention this because anger is the predominant surface emotion in parents, especially in the early weeks and months after they learn of the homosexuality, and naturally their son or daughter feels alienated, rejected, or angry in response. Once the full range of emotions is in place—fear, loss, sadness, hurt, bewilderment, and so forth—and these emotions are being discussed, it is a bit easier for all family members.

The subjective state is mourning, which includes all of the above emotions plus denial ("It's just a phase she's going through"). Parents must mourn the fantasied hopes and dreams that they had for their son or daughter, that is, that he or she would marry and have children. In families in which the gay son or lesbian daughter is an only child, this is harder for parents who longed for a daughter-in-law, or son-in-law, and of course, grandchildren. This longing ceases if their lesbian daughter decides to have a child by a male sexual partner or by artificial insemination. In homes where there are daughters but only one son who is gay, parents mourn because the family name will not be carried on (except of course when/if their daughter keeps her birth name at marriage and her children take her name and not her father's). Parents tend to feel that their work as parents is not completed until their children are grown and married. With a gay son or lesbian daughter, they fear that their "work" will never be done. For many parents, though, this work is completed a few years down the road when their son or daughter is coupled and they have come to accept both the homosexuality and the partner.

Another hardship for parents is related to the stigma that homosexuality carries in our society. They worry about not only their son or daughter's everyday life as a member of a sexual minority group but their future as well. They worry about their son or daughter being alone, or being discriminated against, or being assaulted (we know that gay-bashing and so-called bias crimes are increasing), or about disease—especially AIDS. Many times their worries are seen as intrusive or controlling. This perception can lead to further alienation as their gay son or lesbian daughter pushes for more independence and privacy. When parents and their children can discuss, argue, and debate these issues, it is much easier to resolve them. When the issues can't be discussed, it is very difficult and painful on both sides.

Although the specific determinants of homosexuality remain largely unknown, most gay and lesbian people report feeling inherently different as far back as childhood. For these individuals, their homosexuality feels constitutional, arising from within them. Despite this, there continues to be so much blame associated with homosexuality in our society. Parents blame themselves, or each other, or their child. Society blames the parents and/or the child. Then again, parents may blame society. Whatever the end result, many parents end up feeling terribly closeted themselves, closeted with a shameful secret that their son is gay or their daughter is lesbian. They may tell their very close friends or certain extended family, but maybe not. It is tiring and upsetting for them to continue to respond avoidantly and deceptively to their friends' and family's inquiries about their son's or daughter's singlehood. Parents fear being judged, faulted, or pitied.

Unlike Dr. A, who came to accept his son's gayness partly because he had some medical knowledge from his training and some experience with gay patients from his practice, most doctors have as much difficulty with homosexuality in their family as the general population does. One middle-aged male physician told me, "I've always seen myself as a caring, liberal-minded, and sensitive physician. But I did not realize how much I held my patients' problems at arms length. When my son told me he was gay, I accused him of disgracing our family with his affliction. To this day, I can't believe I said such a horrible thing to him." A woman obstetrician said, "When my daughter Sue confirmed my worst fears that she and Carla were more than roommates, I didn't flinch. I told her I appreciated her honesty and gave her my blessing. What I've never told her is that for three months afterward I got down on my knees every night—me, a card-carrying agnostic—and prayed to God to make her 'normal'—whatever that is! And I prayed for myself for causing it, for divorcing her father, and for working so hard over the years. I'm OK now, and so are they, but I was a mess for a while."

The stress of a son's or daughter's disclosure may produce marital distress or exacerbate underlying and preexisting marital difficulty in couples. Let me give an example of both conflict arising in a current marriage and reactivation of conflict in a previous marriage.

Dr. F's struggle was revealed in his initial overture to me over the phone. His words were, "My wife and I would like to see you. My son has recently told us that he's . . . uh . . . that he's . . . uh . . . my son has recently told us that he's a homosexual. It's—it's been difficult." I arranged for a conjoint visit and learned that their son, Todd, was nineteen years old, living with them, and going to school. Dr. F and his second wife had been married for seven years and had no children of their own. Todd had been living with his mother in another city since his parents' separation ten years earlier; he had come to live with his father and stepmother one year earlier in order to attend college. He volunteered that he was gay one month earlier when his stepmother questioned his withdrawal, irritability, furtive phone calls, and his staying out all night, which was worrying them. A week later he called his mother and told her.

There was tension and hostility on all fronts in this family. Todd was angry and felt unsupported by his father. He felt picked on and babied by his stepmother. He was also adjusting to college, to living with them, and to being separated from his mother. His stepmother was worried about him and his lifestyle; she felt that her husband was being too passive and not showing enough guidance and discipline. His mother was angry at Dr. F. She called him at work and told him that if he had not walked out on her ten years earlier and copped out on his parenting responsibilities, Todd would not be gay. She urged him to have a heart-to-heart talk with Todd, and to get him off to a psychiatrist before it was too late. Needless to say, Dr. F felt bombarded and attacked from all sides. I arranged to meet with all four parties over the next couple of months, individually and in various groupings. These meetings helped to defuse the emotion and to restore harmony. In the end, Todd's father, stepmother, and mother all came to a better understanding and acceptance of his gayness and the partner he met at college.

MAJOR PSYCHIATRIC ILLNESS

In earlier chapters I described some of the ways in which psychiatric illness may affect marriage and how marital difficulties may aggravate a preexisting or accompanying psychiatric disorder. Now I would like to discuss the impact of major psychiatric illness on marriage and family dynamics. Such illnesses usually involve hospitalization and are quite incapacitating, with prolonged periods of time away from medical work or work on a limited schedule. Examples include severe bipolar (manic–depressive) illness, recurrent depression, obsessive–compulsive disorder, schizophrenia, and chemical dependency.

Individuals who suffer from these kinds of illnesses feel a great sense of loss. They have lost their ability to work at an earlier level of high functioning. They also feel a sense of loss of their place in medicine (i.e., they no longer feel a part of mainstream medicine or the sense of collegial interrelating because they are ill so much of the time). These feelings may be accompanied by a loss of stature, recognition, or professional pride because they can no longer practice medicine with fervor or on the same career trajectory. And quite specifically, some may experience a loss of physical function because of various medications they must take, with a range of side effects such as reduced physical stamina, inability to concentrate for long periods, inability to perform surgical procedures, or visual impairment.

Their spouses and children feel tremendous loss as well. They will pine for the person that their mom, dad, husband, or wife used to be. They not only miss that individual and what he or she contributed to their lives (joy, stimulation, influence, or guidance) but simultaneously resent the time spent in the hospital or dysfunction in the home.

Emotional loss like this is sometimes overshadowed by economic loss. Because physicians with severe psychiatric illness miss a lot of time from work or are not able to practice much or any medicine, finances may be tight. There may be socioeconomic decline, with a loss of one's home, neighborhood, friends, ability to afford vacations, or material goods that were once taken for granted. This can result in personal unhappiness, misunderstanding, anger, jealousy, and guilt in all members of the family.

Because of the stigma associated with psychiatric illness, physicians with major psychiatric disorders feel ashamed, and so do their family members. In fact, in some medical families, there may be aggregate shame because of the irrational belief that doctors are not vulnerable to the same illnesses that afflict the rest of humankind. This stigma puts added strain on physicians to "get better fast" or, failing that, deny that anything is wrong. Their families also feel the strain of not being able to tell many of their friends about what is happening at home and why they are feeling out of sorts.

A final note about the loss associated with severe psychiatric illness in physicians and its effects on marriage. These disorders make marriages vulnerable to separation and divorce. And most frightening, there is loss associated with possible or actual suicide in some physicians with these illnesses. Their bereft families are then left to make sense of it all.

This terribly disheartening and sad information about loss must be placed in a wider context. With a greater openness and a more humane understanding in some medical schools and medical communities about psychiatric illness, fewer afflicted individuals and their families feel as isolated and as discriminated against as they might have a generation ago. And with better diagnostic methods and treatment strategies, especially "cleaner" medications, physicians with major psychiatric illness are able to resume work more quickly and to work more effectively. This results in less marital strain and less risk of marital breakdown.

WHEN A SON OR DAUGHTER COMMITS SUICIDE

The death of a child (irrespective of age) is even more painful, and complicated, when that child commits suicide. To my knowledge, there is nothing specific about the kind of grief that physicians and their spouses experience when a son or daughter commits suicide—they agonize no differently, by and large, than laypersons. And I believe that this holds even if the physician parent is a psychiatrist, although there may be more self-blame, as illustrated in this example:

Dr. K was a fifty-five-year-old psychiatrist who came to see me, initially on his own and later with his wife, nine months after his daughter (from his first marriage) committed suicide. Dr. K's chief complaint was: "I'm depressed. My daughter is dead; she killed herself. I can't decide whether to kill myself or not." Words cannot convey the tearful and wrenching emotion of that moment (which I will never forget) when Dr. K poured his heart out to me.

Dr. K went on to tell me about his daughter, a twenty-one-year-old medical student, who was found dead by her roommate. She had taken an overdose of sleeping pills. Although his daughter had not been treated for depression and was not under the care of a psychiatrist, in retrospect it appeared that she had been slipping into a depressed state for about six weeks prior to her death. She had failed two courses and began to withdraw shortly afterward. She began to stay up late to study and then sleep the next day and miss classes. Her roommate started to take lecture notes for her.

Dr. K berated himself for not picking up on his daughter's depression and insisting that she get treatment. She was attending medical school two thousand miles away, however, and they only spoke about twice a month on the phone. Besides, she had not told him about having failed the two courses; she had given him the impression that things were fine. He then wondered if she was not able to be honest with him because, as a physician-father (and a gold medalist in his graduating class), his standards were too high. He also worried if his divorce from his daughter's mother might have contributed in some way to her death. I asked him to explain, and later I was able to reassure him that I did not think so.

My individual psychotherapy work with Dr. K was largely supportive and focused on his grief. His thoughts of suicide gradually receded, and he began to feel stronger again. I insisted that he take a medical leave from his practice of adolescent psychiatry—this kind of work was too close to home, he was not able to assess and treat his patients and their families with enough objectivity, and he had lost all confidence in assessing suicidality in his patients. Later, I had a few conjoint marital sessions with Dr. K and his wife. She had some trouble fully understanding why her husband blamed himself so much. My explanations helped her a lot, and this enabled her to be more supportive of her husband and less confrontative.

Self-blame and "If only I had . . . " attitudes are common in virtually all close family members and friends of someone who commits suicide. Shame is another emotion with which some families struggle (i.e., a sense of embarrassment or humiliation that a member of this family could do such a desperate thing as take his or her own life). Because of so many stereotypical ideas about doctors' families, and the stigma and misconceptions about psychiatric illness in our society, it is not unusual to see shame in doctors' families when a son or daughter commits suicide. Some of these stereotypical ideas are (1) that doctors' kids are all so privileged, there is no reason why they would want to take their lives; (2) that doctors' kids are all screwed up, especially psychiatrists' kids, and that is why they kill themselves; (3) that doctors and their families are up on a pedestal, so if one of their kids commits suicide, then this cannot be true but just a nasty rumor; (4) that parents are to blame when a child commits suicide, and therefore the physician loses his or her credibility as a competent practitioner in his or her community; and (5) that all doctors push their kids academically, therefore he/she killed himself/herself because the parents were disappointed in recent grades or academic standing.

Elsewhere I have written about the propensity to shame, and the ubiquity of shame, in doctors' families.[7] Put this together with some of the above ideas about physicians' lives, and one can see why some medical families even deny or rationalize that their son or daughter's death was self-inflicted. Quite simply, it is just too emotionally overwhelming to begin to consider as a possibility.

Dr. and Mrs. M came for marital therapy because they were fighting all the time and their fourteen-year-old daughter told them that if they didn't get some help, she was leaving! In a sense, she shamed them into coming to see me, because each of them felt that their troubles were not that severe. And they both admitted that they hated the idea of going for professional help.

I asked them to elaborate on their understanding of why they were so tense with each other and why they were fighting so much. There were a lot of problems. Their oldest son, Michael, had been killed in a car accident two years earlier. They both told me how painful this had been for them, but they said that since the first anniversary of his death, they were beginning to get on with their lives. Mrs. M had returned to teaching after many years at home—this called for some acceptance and flexibility on Dr. M's part with his work schedule. Dr. M had seen a number of investments "go under" in the previous few years. He had to declare bankruptcy and this was humiliating for him, in addition to making him feel like a failure. Mrs. M's mother, an elderly widow, was now living with them until they could get her placed in a nursing home. She required assistance and some surveillance because of her failing memory, and her poor hearing drove Dr. M around the bend. More recently, Dr. M had had a brief affair with another doctor in his clinic. Although this relationship was now over, they still worked in the same location and this, understandably, was upsetting to Mrs. M.

I saw the two of them in marital therapy for several months at roughly biweekly intervals. We made some strides, but progress was slow. In one visit, they announced that their daughter had asked to come in to see me on her own, and would I see her? So I did. And what a visit! She began with this: "All of my parents' problems are because Michael committed suicide. I know they haven't told you that, but it's true." She told me that she was seeing a school counselor and that this had helped her a lot to understand what was happening to her family. She talked about a lot of other issues, and the visit ended with her telling me that she was planning to let her parents know that she had told me about the circumstances of Michael's death.

In the next conjoint visit, Dr. M began first. He told me about the long history with Michael. He had a learning disability and poor grades in elementary school. He had problems with drugs in high school and dropped out. He worked at odd jobs and then got arrested for selling marijuana. They sent him away to a treatment center for three months, only to find that he was back on drugs within a month of returning home. After a huge fight with his dad, he took off in his car and several hours later, the police were at the family home: Michael had driven the car off a freeway at eighty miles an hour into an overpass that was under construction. He was killed instantly. "We've never been the same since" were Dr. M's sad words. Mrs. M was silent for a long time (in fact, so was I) and then said, "I think we're ready to do some more work now."

And they were. Things improved a lot now that Michael's death became our focus of therapeutic work. Dr. M had immense guilt about Michael (not *just about what happened the night he committed suicide, but many other frustrating and agonizing misunderstandings and miscommunications over the years), so I had several visits with him alone. Mrs. M also felt that she had let Michael down in many ways, and she needed to talk about this in individual therapy. She had enormous rage at her husband. Some of this anger was recent (about his affair and about the bankruptcy), but most of it was smoldering resentment at him for working so hard over the years and not being around much as a father to Michael when he was a boy. Yet she also felt guilty about these feelings. Her husband had to work long hours because of their high expenses while Michael was growing up (medical school loans had to be repaid, Mrs. M was going to college full-time and was not earning any income then, and Michael's tutoring and special education instruction cost a lot of money). After a course of individual therapy with each of them, I had some more conjoint marital therapy visits, which seemed helpful. A family visit with their daughter confirmed that things were much happier at home. Our work together ended then, and I referred the three of them to a support group for families who have lost a family member to suicide.*

LAWSUITS

The threat of being sued and the reality of a malpractice suit have become part of practicing medicine in North America, particularly in certain specialties. A related, and often no less traumatic, situation occurs when physicians are investigated by their state (or provincial) licensing boards or ethics committees of medical associations or institutions for unprofessional conduct, unusual patterns of practice, fraudulent research, Medicaid or Medicare fraud, and so forth. What are the psychiatric implications of this? How does this kind of stress affect one's marriage?

The psychological stages attendant to being sued are much like the stages of dying or coping with life-threatening illness—shock and disbelief, denial, anger, bargaining, depression, and finally acceptance. Symptoms and behavioral change may include any of the following: irritability, despondency, anxiety, insomnia, embarrassment, frustration, bitterness, loss of work satisfaction, withdrawal from one's family and social activities, emotional distancing from one's patients, hypervigilance at medical work (including self-doubts and ordering unnecessary tests), and premature retirement.[8]

Needless to say, the trauma of being sued rarely spares the spouse and other family members. In fact, in most homes the entire family feels the stress.[9] This is magnified if there has been media coverage of the malpractice or ethical investigation; the family tries to maintain appearances at all costs. If the proceedings have been kept quiet or if the family collusively denies that anything has happened, they may become quite insular, thereby disallowing themselves support from friends and others. In some circles, sued physicians report feeling shunned by their medical colleagues and friends.

Dr. and Mrs. J came to see me for marital therapy. Mrs. J began the first visit with these words: "My husband hates women; they've destroyed him—no, he's allowed them to destroy him. He gave too much the past twenty years. He's used up and bitter. I can't live like this anymore; I hope you can help." Dr. J replied: "I can't argue with her. She's right, I'm burned out. I hate sex, which is OK because I can't get it up anyway. I don't know if I hate women, but if I never had to talk to a woman again in my life that would be fine with me."

Dr. J was a fifty-five-year-old obstetrician and gynecologist, and Mrs. J was a nurse and his office manager. In addition to worries about their five children and residual anxiety about a melanoma that he had had removed eighteen months earlier, Dr. J was most concerned about being sued within the previous three months. There had been a very complicated labor and delivery resulting in a stillborn child. To compound matters, this patient and her family, members of a racial minority group, also were claiming discrimination against them "for inadequate prenatal care." This fact seemed to hurt Dr. J the most, since he not only prided himself on providing competent and compassionate care but also had served many minority families over his long career. The entire case had been the subject of news in their small town's newspaper and radio programming for over a week. Some of Dr. J's patients had left him for the other obstetrician in their community, and he was certain that he was not getting the same number of referrals from family physicians in town.

All of this had caused Dr. J to withdraw into silence and rage. He was not talking to his wife as he once did, nor was he showing any affection or sexual interest in her. Many of his mutterings were condemnatory of women patients, women in general, and the headaches of contemporary medical practice. Mrs. J had tried to be supportive but felt exhausted and frustrated. Because her husband had been sued ten years earlier, she dreaded revisiting that trauma with him and hoped "he would just snap out of it."

Dr. and Mrs. J responded well to marital therapy, which was mainly supportive. They had a healthy, underlying marital infrastructure. I had several more visits with Dr. J on his own, which he found helpful. He really needed to talk about the range of feelings he was having, especially shame and shattered professional self-esteem, so that he could once again feel comfortable and confident with his physician colleagues and friends. He also felt that he had let his family down by "humiliating them in public." A family visit that I scheduled for him, his wife, and their five children was therapeutic and reinforcing for everyone.

In some physicians, a preexisting psychiatric illness may cause impairment that results in a medical or ethical mishap. This illness may have already affected the individual's marriage, leading to severe marital discord, unhappiness, or separation. These added stressors only compound the physician's medical judgment and professional demeanor, putting him or her more at risk for making mistakes. Psychiatric impairment may be due to substance abuse, severe depression, hypomania, or dementia. Emergency or urgent psychiatric assessment and treatment are essential when physicians are struggling with illnesses such as these to prevent harm to patients.

The most serious complication when a physician is sued is suicide.[10] Doctors who are male, are getting older, are separated or divorced, belong to a racial or ethnic minority group, have an associated and severe medical illness, or are chemically dependent are at the greatest risk of taking their own lives if they have been sued. Other factors that make physicians vulnerable to suicide are isolation from peers in medicine, introversion, personal or family history of mood disorder and suicide, and financial hardship. In some branches of medicine like anesthesiology, in which practitioners have easy access to intravenous medications, the risk is even higher.

I strongly recommend that all physicians facing lawsuits be offered psychiatric consultation and involvement in a physicians' support group. I also recommend that hospital departments and medical societies give this subject a higher profile by sponsoring Grand Rounds and seminars on medical malpractice, especially its impact on the individual and his or her family. I urge colleagues and family members of sued physicians to be empathic and supportive; expect irritability in the person; allow ventilation of feelings, over and over again, as necessary; be available; and be reassuring.

DOCTOR–PATIENT BOUNDARY VIOLATIONS

In my work as a psychiatrist and marital therapist, I occasionally see medical couples in which one of the issues is related to the physician-partner's having become sexually involved with a patient (or having been charged with same). Because the most common boundary violation occurs between a male physician and female patient, most of my clinical experience is with these physicians' marriages.

Examples of presenting situations are when a patient complains to medical licensing authorities about her physician's "unprofessional conduct," he is notified, he tells his wife, and a marital crisis ensues; when a couple comes for marital therapy, with the husband having just been charged by the police with sexual assault of a patient and his wife pregnant with their third child; when a couple requests marital therapy because of "stress"—three women patients have complained to the medical licensing board about his "sexually provocative behavior" (which he denies)—and both the man and his wife state that "there are a lot of angry women out there who love to doctor bash"; when a physician falls in love with a patient, either he tells his wife or she finds out, and they come for marital therapy; when, in the course of marital therapy, the couple discloses that they met as doctor and patient, fell in love, and ended their professional relationship; when a physician requests individual therapy, revealing that he is "having an affair" with one of his patients but hasn't told his wife; when a physician calls in a panic after taking a patient in his arms and kissing her passionately, not knowing why he acted so inappropriately and terror-stricken that she might report him; when a physician and his third wife (a former patient of his) come for marital help, new to the community after fleeing another part of the country because of ethical charges against him by two women patients; when a physician with bipolar (manic–depressive) illness stops his lithium and ten days later exposes himself to a female patient during a pelvic exam, and his nurse telephones his wife, who then calls exclaiming, "I can't live with this man anymore—I want out!"; and when a physician and his wife, newly separated, come for marital therapy after he has had his license suspended and becomes suicidal.

The physicians who are most responsive to psychiatric treatment are those who are the most symptomatic. This constitutes the bulk of the physicians who become sexually inappropriate with their patients; very few physicians are sexual predators and recidivists who quite literally "use" their profession to exploit trusting and vulnerable patients. Unrecognized and untreated psychiatric illness or mental conflict is often the primary cause of this type of behavior. The physician's judgment is affected by his or her emotional state, and the normal doctor–patient boundaries become blurred. The physician loses neutrality, clinical objectivity, and measured empathy and can be swept away by powerful thoughts and feelings about the patient. It is very hard for physicians to maintain their usual professional competence and demeanor, especially with certain patients, when they are troubled in their own lives with marital unhappiness, sexual conflict, a new divorce, alcohol abuse, and so forth.

Dr. Z called me requesting marital therapy and asked if I could see him and his wife as quickly as possible, because he had to make a decision whether to separate or not. I saw Dr. and Mrs. Z the following day. Basically the issue was that he was in love with another woman, and he more or less had made up his mind that he was leaving within a few weeks as soon as he could find other accommodations. Mrs. Z was devastated. She was aware that they were not as close as they had been the past couple of years, but she attributed this to her busy schedule with their four children and volunteer work and Dr. Z's hectic work schedule (he was an academic internist on a fast-track career path).

Despite Dr. Z's zeal to end the marriage, he agreed to a course of marital therapy on a very tentative basis. More specifically, he stated that he was prepared to take it a visit at a time and just "play it by ear." He also emphatically stated that he had no intention of giving up his "girlfriend." I agreed to work with the two of them and see what transpired over the next few weeks.

A lot happened. Dr. and Mrs. Z began to talk more together than they had in years. Dr. Z disclosed to his wife that his girlfriend, Ms. G, was actually a patient of his and had been for several years. He had referred her to a colleague a year earlier when they became lovers. Her marriage had ended, and now she was ready to be with Dr. Z. As their communication increased, Dr. and Mrs. Z became closer and more sexually intimate than they had been in a long time. Dr. Z began to reconsider his decision to separate. Shortly thereafter, he ended his relationship with Ms. G abruptly. He refused appeals on Ms. G's part to see her "just one more time," and his marriage continued to improve. I began individual therapy with Dr. Z to help him come to some understanding of his personal and marital dynamics and how he compromised his otherwise impeccable professional standards and became sexually involved with Ms. G.

In the midst of this therapy, as Dr. Z was working on his feelings of remorse, guilt, shame, and self-loathing about this violation of physician–patient boundaries, Ms. G reported him to our local licensing body. He was charged with unprofessional conduct and awaits the outcome of this investigation. Both Dr. and Mrs. Z feel tremendously sorrowful about what has happened and are very fearful of what the outcome of this will be in terms of his medical license and their reputation in the community in which they live and work. Dr. Z regrets that he did not recognize his personal vulnerability earlier (upon reflection, he recalls feeling very lonely in his marriage and somewhat depressed) and that he did not seek professional help when he first began to have loving and erotic thoughts about Ms. G. He also regrets that this subject was never discussed during his training, and that he associated so much stigma with seeking psychiatric help that he delayed going until his situation was quite serious.

When doctors and patients become sexually involved, the fallout can be enormous. Most cases are tragic and extremely upsetting for all parties—the patient and her or his family, the physician and his or her family, and the medical community at large. It is only recently that this subject has received increasing attention in both the professional literature[11-14] and the lay press.[15-16] As a clinician dealing with the mental health implications of boundary violations in the doctor–patient relationship, I believe that the key is prevention. Increasingly, this subject is being taught in medical schools, residency programs, and continuing medical education offerings. I also recommend that psychiatrists become more involved in the investigation of complaints to medical licensing boards and medical society ethics committees. When a physician is being reviewed by a disciplinary body, psychiatric consultation should be suggested and highly urged if the physician seems stressed by the process. It is documented that physicians who lose their medical licenses (or who strongly fear that they might) have a higher risk of suicide than other physicians.[17] They certainly are at risk for depression, substance abuse, and marital discord (or a worsening of these problems if they were present before the alleged offense).

When a physician has more than one complaint against him or her or if the charges are particularly egregious, an assessment by one or more forensic psychiatrists should be ordered to rule out or confirm a personality disorder. I say this because a general psychiatrist not experienced in forensic work may miss major character pathology (including "sexual addiction") in physicians, and there is a chance that these same physicians may abuse more patients in the future if they are not carefully assessed and properly treated.

HIV DISEASE IN MARRIED PHYSICIANS

Few diseases today cause as much dread and anguish as human immunodeficiency virus (HIV), for those individuals who have no symptoms as well as persons whose infection has progressed to full-blown AIDS.[18] Couples who are experiencing marital distress because the man has contracted HIV can benefit enormously from individual, marital, and sometimes family therapy as they cope with the confusion, fear, shame, misunderstanding, and loss that accompany this disease.

Because I have no clinical experience treating female physicians with AIDS, I am restricting my comments here to male physicians. The most common route of infection for married male physicians is by homosexual activity. The physician may have become infected, however, in the course of his work by blood or blood products from a patient with AIDS. Or he may have received transfusions of HIV-contaminated blood or blood products. If the physician has been an intravenous drug user, he may have become infected by that route. Finally, he may have acquired the virus heterosexually from an infected female partner.

What are some of the struggles for the HIV-positive married physician? As I wrote earlier about gay physicians who become HIV-positive, there is continuous mourning. He will mourn his previous good health and anticipated illness, which causes loss of energy and vitality. He may lose his job or his ability to practice medicine as before or at all. He must worry about finances and his ability to provide for the family. There may be concerns about insurance benefits and threats to continued comprehensive coverage for catastrophic illness. There is loss of autonomy and independence and, most important, loss of privacy as one's illness becomes known to medical colleagues, friends, and family (which is often beyond the person's control, given how commonly leaks in confidentiality occur in today's medical centers when physicians become ill).

Another dimension of exposure has to do with sexuality if the married physician is bisexual and has become homosexually infected. He has to come to terms with his bisexuality, which he may have denied or rationalized previously, and to live with his wife's reaction to it, if she had not known before. He has to accept that he has put his wife at risk if they have been sexually active together with no precautions. There is always guilt and shame about this. If there are children, what do they know, and should they be told? Also, what about his parents and other family members? Finally, living with the fact that an increasing number of people, whether caretakers or strangers, know about something as private as one's sexuality requires a degree of dignity and courage that most people never have to test.

What are the issues for the physician's wife? Like her husband, she also will mourn her life as it once was. If she knew nothing of her husband's bisexuality, she must cope with this (i.e., her husband's secret life and now his HIV infection).[19] This means examining her own personal feelings about homosexuality and living with the fact that her husband has not been faithful to her. This sense of betrayal may give her a horrible feeling that her whole marriage has been a sham. She may wonder if her husband ever found her attractive and sexually appealing, and berate and doubt her femininity. Needless to say, marital trust is fractured.

As I mentioned above, she will undergo HIV-antibody testing herself, await the results, and then be retested over the ensuing months. This anxiety is compounded by her anxiety about her husband's professional livelihood and how much longer he may be able to work and contribute to the family income. She will also wonder whether or if they should even remain together as a couple. She may begin to prepare psychologically for early widowhood (and being a single parent, if there are children).

And what about the children? Like their parents, they will also mourn and grapple with the fear and reality of eventually losing their father to AIDS. They will struggle with disclosure to friends of the true nature of their dad's illness. In addition, they have to come to terms with their father's private life and aspects of their parents' marriage— about which many children never know. This is a lot for them to process and for their parents to confront, a fact perhaps most eloquently stated by Susan Sontag: "The illness flushes out an identity that might have remained hidden from neighbors, jobmates, family, friends."[20]

A final comment about treatment. Compassionate and nondiscriminatory care is essential for HIV-positive physicians[21] and their spouses. But because this illness arouses so many feelings in the marital therapist, that individual may need support by colleagues and may need to share the clinical responsibility by involving other therapists. This type of collaborative work, plus regular contact with the infected physician's primary physician or internist, should be well received by the couple.

INTERNATIONAL MEDICAL GRADUATES AND ETHNIC/RACIAL MINORITY MARRIAGES

I touched on stressful issues for international medical graduates (IMGs) in Chapter One. I want to now expand on some of the points I made earlier and to make a few additional comments, especially regarding treatment. This subject is huge, and I can only highlight certain matters.

One of the most common dynamics that I see in troubled marriages of IMGs is isolation or some variant of it. Very often one or both partners miss their families, friends, and aspects of the culture in which they were raised. Sometimes this is mitigated by involvement with other immigrants from their country of origin, but in small medical communities, IMGs may not find others of the same background. Frequently, IMGs have only their spouses for support; this arrangement usually proves to be inadequate and puts inordinate strain on the marriage. If they do not recognize that this is happening, however, they can become very bitter and accusatory, and they may inappropriately conclude that their marriage is over or greatly flawed.

Another common dynamic is economic. Worry about money is one of the most common stressors in all marriages. Because the physician may be delayed in obtaining licensure and board certification in North America, he or she may have a very high debt load. If they are thwarted in establishing a flourishing medical practice because of discrimination against them, IMGs may be further impeded in securing a comfortable income. This may force them to live in a lower-income part of the city and work very long hours to make ends meet. Some married IMG physicians live with their parents or with their spouse's parents. Many are saving and sending money to relatives in their home countries and/or sponsoring the immigration of relatives or friends.

I find that most of these IMGs do not discuss these matters with their North American medical colleagues, who often have no idea how hard they work and the financial strain under which they exist. As one IMG physician said to me: "I don't tell doctors at the clinic that I work an extra job on the weekend; I think they would call me greedy, or a workaholic. I lie and say we all go skiing on the weekends, and pray they don't invite me up to their ski cabins. I've never skied in my life. And I don't tell them what part of the city I live in—I have my pride, too, you know."

A third dynamic, which is related to treatment, is how much IMG physicians may delay seeking help until conditions at home are extreme (i.e., the spouse has attempted suicide, one of the children is symptomatic because of parental conflict, or the physician has become medically ill). Because of cultural differences, some IMGs may be particularly reluctant to obtain psychiatric care. I believe that some delay in seeking assistance is due to the fact that the kind of help that the physician and his/her family need is not often available, or because they perceive that it is not available. Insightful primary care physicians who look after other physicians and their family members will tune into the possibility that matters at home may not be as harmonious as reported. They may gently suggest some type of marital or family therapy. For many IMG physicians, this help is threatening and inappropriate because the therapist does not recognize the sociocultural dynamics that are producing symptoms in the couple. Rapport and trust are never established, and therefore therapy fails. Some couples will try another therapist, but many will not, instead struggling along by themselves.

My final comment pertains not only to IMG physicians and their spouses but also to marriages of ethnic and racial minorities in medicine. When the therapist is of a different "reference group" (whether ethnic, racial, or regional—this occurs frequently in the cultural mosaic of contemporary society) than the physician couple, it is imperative that this fact be recognized and discussed by the therapist in an open and sensitive manner. Even seasoned and well-trained therapists can never fully appreciate the nuances, idiosyncrasies, and subtleties of marital values, roles, expectancies, and communication patterns in couples with unique and rich individual biographies. Only by making this "handicap" explicit and inviting explanation by one or both marriage partners can the therapist earn and gain their respect, trust, and confidence.

CONCLUSION

In this chapter, I have presented some examples of special problems that can affect doctors and their spouses. I have tried to be as specific as possible when it appears that being a physician or a physician's spouse determines how the problems develop, how they manifest themselves, and how they are resolved. Many of these problems are the surface complaints that doctors bring to marital therapy; others underlie the anxiety, tension, and demoralization that characterize the distressed marriage. It is time now to talk about treatment, the subject of the next chapter.

REFERENCES

1. David B. Herzog, Maura Pepose, Dennis K. Norman, and Nancy A. Rigotti, "Eating Disorders and Social Maladjustment in Female Medical Students," *Journal of Nervous and Mental Disease* 173 (December 1985), 734–737.
2. "Anorexia Nervosa," in *Modern Synopsis of Comprehensive Textbook of Psychiatry* (4th ed.), ed. Harold I. Kaplan and Benjamin J. Sadock (Baltimore/London: Williams and Wilkins, 1985), 502.
3. L.K.G. Hsu, "The Etiology of Anorexia Nervosa," in *Annual Progress in Child Psychiatry and Child Development*, ed. S. Chess and A. Thomas (New York: Brunner/Mazel, 1984).
4. Sydney Segal, Margaret Fletcher, and William G. Meekison, "Survey of Bereaved Parents," *Canadian Medical Association Journal* 134 (January 1, 1986), 38–42.
5. Stephen B. Shanfield, G. Andrew H. Benjamin, and Barbara J. Swain, "Parents' Reactions to the Death of an Adult Child from Cancer," *American Journal of Psychiatry* 141 (September 1984), 1092–1094.
6. This case history quoted from Michael F. Myers, "Counseling the Parents of Young Homosexual Male Patients," in *Homosexuality and Psychotherapy*, ed. John C. Gonsiorek (New York: Haworth Press, 1982), 131–143.
7. Michael F. Myers, "Fighting Stigma: How to Help the Doctor's Family," in *Stigma and Mental Illness*, ed. Paul J. Fink and Allan Tasman (Washington, D.C.: American Psychiatric Press, 1992), 139–150.
8. Sara C. Charles, Charlene E. Pyskoty, and Amy Nelson, "Physicians on Trial—Self-reported Reactions to Malpractice Trials," *Western Journal of Medicine* 3 (March 1988), 358–360.
9. Judith S. Samkoff and Gregory K. Gable, "Coping with the Stress of Litigation," *Pennsylvania Medicine* 3 (March 1991), 18–20.
10. Patrick K. Birmingham and Richard J. Ward, "A High-Risk Suicide Group: The Anes-

thesiologist Involved in Litigation," *American Journal of Psychiatry* 142 (October 1985), 1225–1226.

11. Nanette Gartrell, Judith Lewis Herman, Silvia Olarte, Michael Feldstein, and Russell Localio, "Psychiatrist–Patient Sexual Contact: Results of a National Survey. I. Prevalance," *American Journal of Psychiatry* 143 (September 1986), 1126–1131.

12. Glen O. Gabbard, *Sexual Exploitation in Professional Relationships* (Washington, D.C.: American Psychiatric Press, 1989).

13. Council on Ethical and Judicial Affairs, American Medical Association, "Sexual Misconduct in the Practice of Medicine," *Journal of the American Medical Association* 266 (November 20, 1991), 2741–2745.

14. Kathleen Mero Mogul, "Ethics Complaints Against Female Psychiatrists," *American Journal of Psychiatry* 149 (May 1992), 651–653.

15. Melinda Beck, "Sex and Psychotherapy," *Newsweek* (April 13, 1992), 52–57.

16. Megan Rosenfeld, "The Fatal Attraction of Psychiatrist and Patient," *Washington Post* (April 17, 1992), F1–F2.

17. R. Crawshaw, J. A. Bruce, P. L. Eraker, M. Greenbaum, J. E. Lindemann, and D. E. Schmidt, "An Epidemic of Suicide Among Physicians on Probation," *Journal of the American Medical Association* 243 (1980), 1915–1917.

18. Michael F. Myers, "Marital Therapy with HIV-Infected Men and Their Wives," *Psychiatric Annals* 21 (August 1991), 466–470.

19. Michael F. Myers, "Claire and Tom and AIDS," *Canadian Medical Association Journal* 142 (April 1, 1990), 748–749.

20. Susan Sontag, *AIDS and Its Metaphors* (New York: Farrar, Straus, & Giroux, 1988), 24–25.

21. Hacib Aoun, "From the Eye of the Storm, with the Eyes of a Physician," *Annals of Internal Medicine* 116 (February 15, 1992), 335–338.

Chapter Eight

TREATMENT

We have now come to one of the most important topics of this book, namely, treatment. I have organized this section around a question-and-answer format. My aim is practicality for the reader. I also hope to allay anxiety about asking for professional help, to demystify what therapy is all about, and to combat the cynicism that some doctors and/or their spouses harbor toward psychiatric treatment.

WHAT ARE THE WARNING SIGNALS OF A MARRIAGE IN TROUBLE?

All couples have doubts and concerns about their marriages from time to time. People wonder if what they are experiencing is normal and common to all couples. What are the norms and parameters of distress in marriage? "Should I be worried?" is one of the many questions that is asked directly or indirectly by many couples I see in my practice. Some couples come for marital assistance very early, at the first sign of trouble. These people are in the minority. Many have been married before and do not want to reexperience marital unhappiness or divorce. But most couples who come for marital therapy are quite distressed and have had problems a long time. They frequently say, "I wish we had come five years ago," or a variant thereof.

So what should you look for in alerting yourself to problems? In the earlier chapters I divided problem areas according to various groupings—medical students, resident physicians, women physicians, and so forth. Some of the case studies that I cited contain verbatim statements of feeling states that may strike a familiar chord. The best clue to possible marital unrest is the presence of subjective symptoms, that is, feelings of tension and anxiety, insomnia, change of appetite, irritability, angry outbursts, and unhappiness. You may notice an increase in physical symptoms (e.g., headaches, chest pain, upset stomach, back pain, or a flare-up of preexisting psychosomatic disorders such as peptic ulcer disease, asthma, migraine, or rheumatoid arthritis). Most notably, you must pay attention to an increase in alcohol consumption or recreational drug usage. Self-medicating with tranquilizers or painkillers is another warning signal. Persistent and serious fantasies of separation that last for weeks or months are also indicative of marital unhappiness.

Even if you have none of these symptoms yourself, you must pay attention to these or similar changes in your spouse. It is not unusual for only one member of a couple to manifest symptoms of a marital problem or for one member to feel only secondarily affected by the distress of the other. "I'm very happy with our marriage. The only time I get upset is when my wife is unhappy," stated one physician. In some families, the parents feel fine, but it is their child who is symptomatic with frequent stomachaches, temper tantrums, aggressive behavior, or bed-wetting. The child is the identified patient, the beacon of an underlying and unrecognized marital problem. If these parents express unhappiness, it is not with each other, it is with the child.

In addition to individual symptoms, you and your spouse may exhibit marital symptoms. You may bicker with each other or nitpick over many if not most matters of mutual concern. Or you may find yourselves arguing a lot, more than usual, and without resolution of the argument. The same issues may arise over and over again. Arguing may accelerate to fighting that becomes verbally violent with insults, name-calling, and threats. If you are a man, you are more prone to physical violence when angry, that is, pushing, slapping, or hitting your wife, than to being hit yourself. If you are not the type to discharge aggression or angry feelings directly, you may retreat into silence and emotional withholding. You may also withdraw physically from your spouse; you no longer make affectionate gestures or want affection. You no longer feel sexually interested in or aroused by your spouse. Your communication with each other is icy, wooden, or formal.

There are other marital symptoms: You may find yourself actively avoiding your spouse, not wanting to do anything together, not wanting to share or discuss anything except mundane everyday happenings. When you socialize it is always with other individuals, couples, or family; in other words, you never go out just as a couple alone together. You find you have nothing to say to each other while alone together—or fear you will have nothing to say. You find your lives together becoming increasingly parallel or divergent; the areas of overlap and shared activity and purpose (except the children) become fewer and fewer. You begin to feel that your spouse is no longer your best friend.

At this time or earlier you may find yourself involved in an extramarital relationship. In fact, for many doctors or their spouses, the earlier-mentioned feelings, thoughts, or symptoms do not happen or become clear until they have met someone else and become reflective about their marriage. Being involved with someone else is usually a mixed blessing—it can be both soothing and frightening, exhilarating and depressing, clarifying and confusing, energizing and exhausting. It will bring things to a head for you and prompt decision making: whether to end the affair and remain in your marriage, whether to end your marriage and continue in the new relationship, whether to try to maintain both the outside relationship and the marriage, or whether to leave both relationships and be on your own. You may come to these decisions and implement them with or without professional help.

The following is an example of a couple who came for help early:

Pam and Harold were both aged thirty-three and had been married for five years when they came for help. Pam was a nurse, six months pregnant and working part-time; Harold was a family physician. They had a two-year-old son at home. Neither had been married before.

Pam was the initiator of marital help (Harold had no complaints). Her chief complaint was, "Our communication is slipping." She went on to elaborate: "We don't talk like we used to—either as frequently or as openly. We are both very busy and don't see each other as much as before. Most of our interaction is around Josh, our son—by the time he's in bed, we're beat and ready for bed ourselves. I've also noticed that we get short with each other, a lot actually, and that's not conducive to relaxed, intimate talk." Basically Harold agreed with these and many other observations of Pam's, but he couldn't understand why she was "making a federal case out of it and going to see a shrink." She went on to make several comments that helped Harold to appreciate her concern. She stated that she had attempted to discuss these matters several times with him and found him dismissive. She told Harold that she wanted to have her parents look after Josh for a weekend while they went away as a couple. He responded that they couldn't afford it. She admitted that she was anxious about their communication possibly worsening with the added responsibility of their second child. A couple of their friends, including Harold's partner in his medical practice, recently separated, and this frightened her. Finally, Harold's parents (both doctors) had separated when he was a teenager after many years of strife and melancholy in the home—she didn't want this.

Then there is this example of a couple who came for help much later:

Lucy, an ear, nose, and throat specialist, was also the mother of children aged six, eight, and ten. She came to see me two weeks after asking her husband, Jim, a general surgeon, to leave. She came because of her mood, wondering if it was normal to feel depressed "at a time like this." Actually she was coping extremely well under the circumstances. Her husband was involved with another woman; this relationship had begun shortly before their separation. Lucy felt confused. She admitted that their marriage had been strained for years, that she wasn't sure if she loved Jim, or if she wanted to even allow herself to entertain the possibility of marital therapy then or later. She knew one thing—that she was furious at her husband for becoming involved with someone else so quickly, that she felt rejected, used, and humiliated. She didn't know if she could ever trust or respect him again. She respected him, though, as a father and didn't want to jeopardize or undermine his relationship with their children.

I set up a visit with Jim, whose opening words were, "We, Lucy and I, should have been here years ago." He also felt confused and unsure of his actions and motives. He admitted that he still loved Lucy in many ways but that he was also in love with Alice, the woman whom he had recently met. Being separated bothered him. It felt wrong to him as a husband and father not to be in an intact family. He missed daily contact with his children and felt guilty for, in his words, "breaking up the home and putting Lucy and the kids through all of this." He also expressed a lot of anxiety about being on his own for the first time in many years and adjusting to living in an apartment again.

WHAT CAN I DO ON MY OWN WITHOUT MARITAL THERAPY?

Having identified some of the personal and interpersonal warning signals of marital difficulty, there are many things that you alone and you and your spouse together can do to ease the difficulty or to eradicate it completely. By doing that, you may obviate the need for marital therapy then or later. On the other hand, there are some problems that are so delicate or so deeply fundamental that they are impossible to discuss together without severely hurting or enraging one another. These are best handled with the assistance of a trained professional.

So what can you do on your own? Recognizing and accepting that there is a problem is the first step to a solution. This is easier said than done. There are at least two stages: labeling the unpleasant feeling state or the negative interaction as a problem, and then acknowledging one's part in the creation or reinforcement of that situation.

Dr. V and Mrs. V had not made love for six months. Both felt that this was a problem that needed discussion. Dr. V volunteered that he had not been feeling very interested in sex. He was preoccupied with medicolegal matters since being sued by a patient several months earlier. Mrs. V stated that she had noticed his preoccupation and, although feeling her normal level of sexual desire, decided not to bring it up for fear of pressuring him. Dr. V responded that he did not know that and that he had begun to wonder about her sexual interest. He also requested that she initiate sex more, that his own sexual lethargy was probably more apparent than real. She agreed to this easily, and soon they were making love again at their regular frequency.

Would that all marital issues were so simple! Unfortunately, many couples get bogged down in one of these stages. One person perceives a problem, but the other does not. Sometimes this difference in perception is present the first time the matter is broached and becomes more obvious or agreed upon the second or third time, perhaps weeks or months later. How a perceived problem is raised is critical. If you bring up a concern in a harshly dogmatic or accusatory way, you are almost guaranteeing that the concern will be denied or argued (e.g., "You never talk to me anymore," "You always interrupt me when I speak," or "You're just like your father"—distant, stubborn, argumentative, sexist, etc.). Using the first person plural, being tentative, and reporting feelings works better (e.g., "We don't seem to talk as easily anymore," or "I feel unhappy that we can't talk like we used to").

Other couples may take years to agree on the presence of problems or the need for outside help. One of the most common statements I hear in my practice is, "I wanted to come for help a year ago, but my husband refused." The duration of this may be as long as twenty or more years in some couples. Occasionally it is the wife who is reluctant to come for help.

Even when you can both agree that there is a problem, it may be difficult for you to see or acknowledge the second stage, that is, your part in creating and maintaining the problem. It is always easier to "put it out there," to see one's partner's role in it or to attribute all responsibility or blame to one's partner. Here are common laments: "My husband works too hard." "My wife yells constantly." "My husband drinks too much." "My wife drinks too much." "My husband's never been affectionate." "My wife demands affection." These sample complaints all elicit a defensive response in the recipient, which then precludes any further discussion of the matter. Nobody likes to hear that he or she drinks too much, or that he or she has a sexual problem!

What else can two people do on their own to improve things without seeking professional help? Try to really listen to your spouse, understand that the concerns are being aired in good faith, that he or she is trustworthy and not trying to render you "one down." If you can really trust your spouse, then you can accept that the complaint is sincere. Although trust is fundamental, and the bedrock of a healthy marriage, it waxes and wanes in most marriages from time to time. It is hard to communicate honestly and openly when trust is fractured or suspect. Further, it is normal to feel defensive about many, if not most, of one's liabilities and insecurities. Accept that both you and your spouse will feel defensive when trying to communicate on many issues, especially the more sensitive ones. Admit this to each other. Your defensiveness should diminish in time.

A brief word to male doctors and husbands of female doctors. As I have stated in earlier chapters, most women monitor the functional state of their marriages. They become concerned when communication breaks down, they watch their and their husband's degree of happiness in the marriage, and they read about marriage and how to keep relationships alive and healthy. Therefore, listen to your wives! They are not overreacting or just picking on you. Nor are they blaming you for all the marital difficulty. Unfortunately, by the time many husbands come for therapy with their wives, it appears this way. All that is visible is anger on both sides. He is angry that they cannot solve things themselves and feels threatened by her; she is angry that he took so long to consent to professional help. Also, her anger may seem like total condemnation of her husband and denial of her own part in the marital trouble. Such one-sidedness is rare.

Accept that you are human and therefore, like all married people, you are vulnerable to marital distress from time to time. You and your spouse may be able to solve most of your differences yourselves, but there may be some that are irresolvable and do not go away. Also, keep in mind that in a marriage there are times that may be more stressful (e.g., during residency,[1] or during certain types of residencies or rotations that have a lot of on-call and long working days). Although this is not clearly documented, there are some specialties in medicine, especially surgery and the surgical subspecialties, that are so labor-intensive that they affect spouses and children, to say nothing of the eventual mental health pressures on the doctors themselves.

Pay attention to personal and familial factors. If you suffer from depression, alcoholism, or dependency on other drugs, you are at greater risk for marital difficulty, separation, and divorce. Also, if your parents have divorced, you may be more prone to marital breakdown yourself. The reasons for this are far from clear; it is certainly not a direct cause-and-effect relationship. Most couples divorcing today grew up in intact homes, and not all offspring of a divorced couple go on to divorce themselves. I mention these facts not to be an alarmist but to heighten the consciousness of people about their marital health.

This brings me to my next point. You must recognize and accept that all marriages require attention and work. I can suggest other requirements, too: care, time, thought, consideration, patience, sacrifice, nurturance, and grooming, among others. Reading this book, and taking in other forms of information, is a concrete example of the type of attention needed.

Make an effort to set aside time as a couple on a regular basis—at least weekly—for talk, relaxation, romance, and possibly sex. I say "possibly sex" because it does not always follow from the other activities; and in most marriages sexual activity does not exist in isolation. You can't have healthy and mutually satisfying sex without verbal and emotional closeness. Observe yourself over a period of a few weeks to see if you do set aside the time for togetherness. Note if you "forget" to do it, or reply that you've "been too busy" to do it. Also note if you actively avoid setting the time aside. Do not conclude that you don't care, or concede to your spouse's allegation that you don't care—at least not yet. This avoidance may not really be a lack of caring but a fear. It may be a fear of getting into a fight or a fear of intimacy or a fear of emptiness—that you have nothing to say to each other or an awkwardness at being alone together.

I also recommend that you try to get out together as a couple once a week (or at least once in two weeks). Many couples find that they have their best talks outside of the home because there are no interruptions (the phone ringing, someone coming to the door, the children awakening, etc.). This time together must be protected, so it is wise to mark it on the calendar and not to let other commitments intrude.

Attempting what I am suggesting may not come easy. These efforts, simple as they sound, are really quite foreign to most people; they may be hard to squeeze into the busy schedule of a doctor's life, especially when there are small children and a lot of other commitments to extended family, and friends, and community work to consider. It is precisely at this phase of the marital life cycle, when people are especially busy with careers and small children, that it is essential to have one-to-one time together as a couple. It is very easy to lose sight of each other as best friends, companions, and lovers and begin to interact only as parents of shared children. Also, most physicians have not witnessed this relationship primacy that I am suggesting in their families of origin. Nor have they learned it in school, including medical school and residency!

Cultivate other couples as close and trusted friends. They will not only enhance one's socialization experience, but they will be there to share experiences common to all married couples in general and to medical couples in particular. Other couples can be an invaluable source of comfort, support, and reassurance at times of marital distress. Couples who are a bit older, or who have been together longer, or who have experienced and survived troubles similar to your own can also serve as role models. Male doctors tend to underestimate the importance of couple friends, and maybe even personal male friends, until they find themselves in a crisis. It may be only then that they come to value the presence and solace of their friends.

Something else that you can do on your own without professional help is to start working on whatever the problem is, once it is identified by you or your spouse. This is possible for some problems; a conscious, deliberate, intentional perseverance will work. Steps you may take include working fewer hours, learning to say no to more work, returning to work part-time instead of full-time, drinking less or stopping altogether, postponing a residency or fellowship, or booking a vacation. The underlying motive here is that you and your spouse agree that these are indeed problems and there is something to be gained (e.g., marital harmony) by changing them. Unfortunately, many couples argue about their identified problems without reaching a consensus. Conflicts over power result, and problem behaviors remain unchanged.

You and your spouse may want to try a marital enrichment experience available in your community. Generally, these meetings are for marriage enhancement only and not for couples with severe problems. They are predicated on the premise that all marriages can use renewal, growth, and new learning. Both participants are assumed to be willing and interested. The functions are usually scheduled as a weekend encounter with other couples. Some groups meet for several weeks for a couple of hours. Most, but not all, are sponsored by the major religions. Those that are spiritually inspired will vary a great deal in the role that religious dogma plays in the format. I state this because couples who are less religiously inclined frequently balk at the notion of attending any marital workshop that is nonsecular in origin.

Regardless of what they are called, these groups usually use a workshop format. These "workshops" are often a mix of didactic instruction on communication theory and experiential work that allows you to try out what you've heard and read. Learning to use and practice techniques such as rephrasing comments, paraphrasing, active listening, keeping statements brief, and reporting feelings are commonly part of the format. Role-playing, wherein you take your spouse's part in a marital dialogue, is an effective tool that allows you to begin to appreciate your spouse's position. Some workshops have themes more specific than general communication, for example, effective parenting, coping with extended family, understanding stepfamilies, and improving sexual expression in marriage.

One word of warning about Marriage Encounter, a church-sponsored marriage enrichment program. Several studies on its potential hazards have been made by Doherty, Lester, and Leigh.[2] These authors, although hampered by lack of cooperation from Worldwide, one of the two rival branches of Marriage Encounter, have found that a small percentage of the couples that they interviewed reported negative effects after the weekend. Most of these couples were highly maritally distressed before the experience. The authors' main recommendation is a more rigorous screening procedure to discourage people with psychiatric conditions and/or severe marital distress from attending Marriage Encounter.

Finally, you may want to read books about marriage. Once again, I find women more interested in reading about marriage. Usually, they come across an interesting article in a magazine or find a book that is helpful; they ask their husband to read it and set it aside for him. Days and weeks pass without comment from him until his wife brings it up. Usually he hasn't read it and makes an excuse; deep inside he really is not that interested. It would have been much simpler and clearer had he said that he wasn't interested in the beginning. It doesn't necessarily mean that he does not care, unless this is part of a whole constellation of avoidant moves. It could simply mean that reading is not his way to work at his marriage.

WHEN SHOULD WE SEEK PROFESSIONAL HELP?

My advice about when to seek professional help is that you try some of the suggestions discussed above and give yourselves at least a few weeks to a few months to work on changing things. You should be able to tell if things are beginning to feel calmer or happier, or if communication and problem solving seem easier. Many couples tell me that there is a pattern to their distress, that their problems are cyclical and recurrent. Consequently, they do not trust that they have truly improved or learned new ways of living together until a sufficient period of time has passed and they are still feeling fine.

If things do not seem to be getting better or change is extremely slow or equivocal, do not despair. And do not associate seeking professional help with failure. There are many problems that on the surface seem simple and straightforward but, because of other variables (some of which are beyond awareness or unconscious), are not easily resolved. You may find that you and your spouse are going around in circles, or becoming entangled and embroiled in issues from which you cannot see your way clear. It may mean that the problem is a tip-of-the-iceberg phenomenon with long-standing historical dimensions not immediately visible except to the eye of a trained observer and experienced therapist.

You may be struggling with other problems that you long ago defined as being difficult and complicated. They may be ones that you once tried to discuss and work through, but without success. You or your partner felt hurt, or angry, or attacked, or betrayed, and this precluded further attempts at resolution. Sexual complaints are common to the group of problems that are hard to discuss; other concerns are the disciplining of biological children in stepfamilies, excessive drinking in one partner, unresolved feelings over a previous affair, and changing sex roles and attitudes around the home. These are much more easily approached with the guidance and assistance of a marital therapist.

If things at home are escalating rapidly into severe tension, arguments, verbal and physical violence, and threats of separation, try to arrange for an early visit with a therapist. Just having come to a decision to seek professional help, even if you have to wait a while for the appointment, usually eases tension a bit at home and makes it possible to get along. If you and your spouse have more or less decided to separate, I still urge you to book a consultation visit with a marital therapist. His or her experienced counsel will assist you in affirming your decision or in delaying a bit. Sometimes trial marital therapy is illuminating: You may be overreacting to your disenchantment with each other; separating hastily is not the solution or it may be premature. The therapist may urge you to slow down your plans to separate; in the process of doing this, mutual anger and frustration may be discharged, some positive feelings for each other may return, and separation may be postponed or later found unnecessary. Even if separation is inevitable, slowing it down, if possible, gives all of you time to prepare for it, both physically—finding new accommodations, sorting out shared possessions and furnishings, saving money—and psychologically. It gives you more time to grieve and work through all of the many feelings I described in Chapter Five. Also, seeing a marital therapist when deciding to separate validates your decision to live apart; it affirms that the marriage cannot be worked on and that the act of separating is indeed real.

WHAT ARE THE BENEFITS OF OUTSIDE HELP?

There are at least five advantages in requesting and receiving outside help.

TALKING TO A PROFESSIONAL PERSON

For something as important as one's marriage, one's mental health, and the mental health of one's family members, it is wise to consult a professional person. Apart from being trained in a discipline, having the proper knowledge base, and being experienced in treating couples in distress, your therapist should also be objective and neutral without being cold or mechanical. This objectivity is something friends and family cannot provide because of their varying emotional attachments to one or both of you. Your therapist should also be a keen observer and diagnostician. These skills include seeing the issues that are not clear to you and your spouse, sifting through confusing and contradictory communications, facilitating emotional expression at times and putting a lid on it at other times, and most importantly, determining when or if you or your spouse is in need of more intensive treatment, such as individual therapy and/or medication.

A well-trained professional should be able to offer assistance, guidance, and hope. I do not mean hope in the narrow sense, that the two of you will stay together, but in a more general sense, that you will each get through this very difficult time in your lives whether you remain together or not. All good therapy is based on the premise of trust, and you should be able to believe completely that your therapist has your best interests at heart. Therapy does not include taking your side against your spouse or taking your spouse's side against you. If or when you feel this is occurring you must bring it up directly with your therapist, for if it persists, treatment will not work.

There is something distinctly advantageous to forming a working relationship with your therapist. The therapeutic relationship is very different than a personal friendship, although it may encompass aspects of friendship such as mutual respectfulness, warmth, liking each other, and, of course, trust. Here are statements I commonly hear in my work with couples: "We like coming here to talk these things out because we don't have to worry about wearing out and alienating our friends." "Our friends are wonderful and very supportive, but most of them take my side against my husband (or wife)." "You seem to be the only one who understands why we're not divorced." "You haven't said anything that we didn't really know, but because you're a professional, I find that we listen to you." "I like the fact that we don't know you personally or run into you socially. I feel I can really be honest and open here without fearing judgment."

EXPEDITING CHANGE

Working with a third person who is trained, experienced, and out-side your everyday life speeds up the process of beginning to feel better again, thinking more clearly, becoming more decisive, and taking action. This change in approach can be extremely important and wel-come when you are bogged down in marital worries, are very ambiva-lent about what to do, or are paralyzed into inactivity by feelings of guilt and despondency. In most cases, you will be able to tell when or if you are stuck or at a stalemate with each other. "We've been spinning our wheels for six months—I know we love each other and want to make this work, but at the moment we can't discuss anything except the weather without bickering," said a thirty-six-year-old family physician hoping to get his marriage functioning again after an extramarital affair.

SHARING RESPONSIBILITY WITH ANOTHER PERSON

It helps to be able to transfer some of the responsibility for your marriage onto someone else for a while. I don't mean complete respon-sibility, which would be a false premise because ultimately you bear the responsibility for your marriage anyway. This transfer is more subtle and has to do with at least two factors: first, you and your spouse feel overwhelmed or confused or powerless with your relationship, and second, you perceive hope, strength, and trust in your therapist. This perception enables you to let go a little or a lot, depending on many variables: your ages, duration of your marriage, degree of your stress together, age of your therapist, sex of your therapist, therapeutic style of your therapist, and whether you are in short-term or long-term therapy.

Laura and Brad were senior medical students; both were twenty-six years old. They had been married for three years when they came for marital therapy. They had problems in many areas: they had no money, Brad was in academic difficulty, their sexual relationship was infrequent and unfulfilling to each of them, Brad's divorced mother was overly dependent on them, and Laura was struggling with unresolved feelings about a therapeutic abortion three months previously. Neither had lived away from their families before they got married. As much as they loved each other, they also felt enormous responsibility for the other, coupled with resentment, and a need for space. Therapy included a combination of conjoint and individual work, to which they responded well. I was touched by Brad's concluding words in our final visit: "Thanks for letting us dump all this crap on you—we would never have made it without your big shoulders."

In another instance:

Janice and Jim had been married for twelve years. They had two sons, six and eight years of age, when they came for therapy. They were both family physicians in the same group practice. The major concerns were Jim's temper, his abuse of alcohol, and Janice's complete disinterest in sex. Although Jim had abstained from alcohol for three months, Janice remained quite unhappy and wanted to separate, perhaps not permanently but for at least six months. Jim was completely against this and only wanted to work on the marriage. Janice's feelings were strong and her mind was made up; she stated that she was prepared to leave their home and take an apartment with the children if Jim would not consider leaving himself. By the third conjoint visit with me, Jim had agreed, albeit unhappily, to take an apartment himself. Both Jim and Janice had many questions regarding the separation—how and when to tell the children, how to arrange visitation, when to seek legal counsel, questions about mediation, and so forth. Their collective statement to me was poignant: "We're counting on you. It's not everyday we go through this process—it's very scary."

ALLEVIATING GUILT

Most doctors and/or their spouses with marital troubles feel very guilty, particularly in situations when there are children, especially young children; when there is a lot of tension, arguing, and fighting in the presence of or within earshot of the children; when there are threats of separation or a decision to separate; and when only one partner wants the separation, whether the couple has children or not.

When your guilt is strong or overwhelming it is very helpful to talk with a therapist. Not only will it feel better to talk about it and "get it off your chest," so to speak, it helps to have your predicament validated and your actions understood. Further, your therapist will be working with the two of you to assist in whatever manner is indicated: to help decrease the tension and fighting at home, to suggest ways of your talking with and reassuring the children that something is being done, and to meet with the children if necessary. Even the act of reaching out for professional help and attempting marital therapy is helpful in reducing your guilt if you go on to separate. It will support your decision to live apart as a correct one, an inevitable one, and a permissible one. The feeling is something like, "We've tried everything, including marital therapy and nothing has worked. It's OK to separate."

IT WORKS!

The evidence that therapy is helpful when you are maritally distressed is not just impressionistic but also empirical.[3,4] It is particularly helpful to have someone outside your situation with clear vision to see what is going on, to act as a guide and facilitator, and to provide some sense of hope. You should begin to feel better again, perhaps not immediately, but certainly after a few visits.

Having said this, there are some couples whose situation may feel worse before it gets better. This is because there are old or underlying issues that need resolution before you can move on to your present-day issues. Your therapist should be alert to this possibility and explain it to you. Also, it is wise to remember that the focus in therapy is on the problems, what is *not* working as opposed to what is working. Consequently, you must not lose sight of the fact that in many ways, you and your spouse get along very well and are happy together. The exception of course is if your marital issues are irreconcilable, if there is very little holding the two of you together, and separation cannot be prevented.

WHAT KIND OF PROFESSIONAL HELP IS INDICATED?

I want to address this question in two ways: (1) What help do two people in the general population who are maritally distressed need, and who can provide it? (2) What help do medical couples who are maritally distressed need, and who can provide it? For some couples, what is important is not so much whether one or both are doctors but the specific nature of their marital problem(s). For example, their main complaint may be a sexual dysfunction, bisexuality in one of them, alcoholism, stepfamily conflicts, or physical violence. In large cities, they may be best to consult a marital therapist subspecialized in one of these fields. Other couples may have a mixed bag of concerns well within the expertise of a wide range of marital therapists: Dual career couples, whether both are doctors or not, will want to ensure that whomever they consult is experienced and bias-free in his or her approach to married couples.

In smaller communities, there may be a problem of treatment discrepancy; that is, what is needed and indicated in your case is not available. You may have to travel to a nearby urban center for the specific and/or perhaps more specialized care that you need. Some of you, to protect your privacy, will prefer to seek help outside your community anyway; in other words, help is available locally, but you know all of the therapists personally or professionally, or you don't necessarily like, trust, or respect them.

When you begin to recognize and accept that you and your spouse are unable to work out your conflicts yourselves and are considering seeing a marital therapist, try to discuss it if possible. It is important to consider not just your own needs and preferences but also your spouse's. What do each of you want from a therapist? Are your goals similar or quite different? Would your spouse accept or reject the therapist you would like to see? With whom might your spouse be most comfortable or trusting? What can you do, if anything, to make this decision and process less threatening for yourself and for your spouse?

This is easier said than done. Many couples attempt to discuss these likes and dislikes but get nowhere. Their lack of agreement is understandable and may beg the question. "If we were able to communicate that easily, we wouldn't need to see a therapist!" is a fitting response. I see many couples in my practice whose decision was made unilaterally, and one partner feels coerced and bullied into treatment. This has been the modus operandi in many aspects of their relationship and quickly becomes one of the problems to work on in therapy. I also see individuals who know they have a marital problem but have been unsuccessful in getting their spouse to come in with them. Sometimes I am successful in suggesting new approaches to try with reluctant, frightened, and unwilling spouses.

I would like now to mention briefly the four most common professions that do marital therapy.

FAMILY PHYSICIANS

Although somewhat regionally distributed throughout North America, family physicians are the first ones to whom many maritally distressed couples turn. Elsewhere I have written about the common marital problems that couples bring to their family physicians, methods of assessment, and treatment guidelines.[5] Even when family doctors themselves do not do marital therapy, they will be called upon to refer their patients to someone who does.

It is not known how often family doctors treat couples wherein one or both partners are doctors themselves. It is probably not common, given that so many doctors do not even have a family physician. If they do have one, they may not have cultivated an intimate doctor–patient relationship with him or her. They may tend instead to use their family doctor as a resource person for referral to specialists. In many situations, doctors' spouses go to their family doctors with marital troubles, but unfortunately their complaints do not always get thoroughly assessed and investigated.

Here is a not uncommon example:

> *Mrs. Green complained to her family physician, Dr. Armstrong, that she was feeling depressed and anxious about her marriage. She complained that she and her husband, a family physician, were fighting a lot, especially about his increasing use of alcohol. Recently, her husband had struck her a couple of times; this behavior was out of character for him. Dr. Armstrong told her that family medicine is very stressful and prescribed a tranquilizer for her! She asked if he would see her husband and talk to him, but he avoided the question. Three months later, she told the same story to her internist, a regular golf partner of her husband's. He replied that her husband's drinking couldn't be that bad, because he'd never noticed excessive drinking when he was with him. Six months later her husband was charged with impaired driving. At this point, she called the physicians' aid hotline (of their local impaired-physicians' committee), which intervened by getting her husband detoxified and then into an alcohol treatment program. The addiction medicine specialist in turn referred Dr. and Mrs. Green to me for marital therapy.*

What this example illustrates is the conspiracy of silence surrounding personal and marital difficulty in the physician. Patients' complaints, whether they are by doctors or their family members, must be taken seriously. There are many reasons, well documented in the published literature of the past twenty years, for inactivity on the treating physician's part—denial of troubles in doctor colleagues, embarrassment, guilt, timidity in approaching the symptomatic doctor, and simple ignorance. More doctors in the 1990s are better educated on this subject, and we are beginning to see some changes.

I suggest that those of you who have a family physician speak to him or her if you are worried about your marriage. Your family physician should be there to listen, to gauge the severity of your concerns, to rule out any complicating or additional problems, to provide comfort, and to discuss treatment. If you are the spouse of a physician, make sure that your husband or wife is interviewed, especially if you sense that both your doctor and your spouse are avoiding it!

RELIGIOUS COUNSELORS

A significant number of people consult their minister, priest, rabbi, or other spiritual leader about marital concerns. They may go individually or together; they may receive specific counseling for their difficulties or a recommendation to seek counseling elsewhere, depending on their needs and the training of their religious advisor. How commonly doctors approach the clergy about their marital concerns is not known.

I always ask medical couples who are religious and actively practicing their religion whether they have spoken to their minister, priest, or spiritual advisor. I am surprised how often couples reject nonsecular counseling as something they've never considered and never would. The reasons vary: "This is too personal," "He's not trained in counseling," "I don't want a religious trip laid on me," "We know him too well," "I couldn't tell my troubles to him," or "He's pretty traditional and quite sexist" are common responses. Couples who are separated or contemplating separation fear they will receive a lecture on the sanctity of marriage and using divorce as a way of avoiding personal, family, and social responsibilities.

On the other hand, some couples may have spoken to religious counselors about marital troubles and found them very helpful. Those who are divorced may have been helped before, during, or after by a minister, priest, or member of the clergy. It really depends a great deal on what religion the couple belongs to, how conservative or liberal its dogma is, the couple's specific and unique marital dynamics, and their spiritual leader's understanding, training, and experience in his or her work. Catholic physicians and their spouses who are divorcing may need counseling to learn about annulment. Orthodox Jewish doctors and spouses may need to discuss the "get," that is, the process in Jewish law by which the husband "grants" the divorce and the wife "receives" it.

NONMEDICAL THERAPISTS

By nonmedical therapists I mean the bulk of professionals who do marital therapy, usually psychologists and social workers, and occasionally people with degrees in education. Training requirements vary, but the best nonmedical therapists will have a master's or doctorate degree from a major university, will be licensed, and will be registered with the local branch of their national professional association in their community. Some will have done further training and course work in marital and family therapy and will belong to one or more of the major national and international organizations, such as the American Association for Marriage and Family Therapy, the American Family Therapy Association, or the American Orthopsychiatric Association. Ask your therapist what his or her credentials are regarding training and membership in professional associations and societies.

As a physician you may prefer to see a nonmedical therapist, and there are many reasons for this. You may fear that a physician therapist (family doctor or psychiatrist) will tell you that your marital problems are "normal" in medical marriages—and not worthy of his or her time or attention. In other words, you worry that you will be dismissed or not taken seriously. You may feel that in your community the medical therapists are not as well trained or as experienced as the nonmedical therapists in marital work. You may fear that a physician therapist, especially a psychiatrist, will label you with a psychiatric diagnosis, that he or she will be biomedically biased and disease oriented. And you may fear being treated with medication, not marital therapy. These labeling and medication concerns will be especially pronounced if you did suffer from a major psychiatric illness at one time, requiring medication and/or hospitalization, and the treatment or experience with the psychiatrist did not go well. If your problem with alcohol or drugs is complicating your marital life, you may fear that a physician therapist, but not a psychologist or social worker, would report you to your local medical society or licensing body.

There are two other common fears in physicians about receiving marital therapy (and other kinds of therapy) from psychiatrists. Some physicians fear (erroneously) that a psychiatrist would report them to the National Practitioner Data Bank. The NPDB opened on September 1, 1990, to monitor medical incompetence.[6] What are reported are malpractice charges and payments and adverse actions against physicians' licenses to practice medicine; seeking psychiatric care is not reportable. A second source of anxiety in physicians who seek marital therapy by a psychiatrist has to do with disability insurance—that is, if or when a physician later applies for disability insurance (or applies to increase a preexisting type of insurance), he or she will be asked to give consent for release of information regarding having sought earlier psychiatric treatment. A marital problem is not a psychiatric diagnosis, but if there was an associated illness (e.g., substance abuse, depression, or panic disorder) that was treated, the psychiatrist must state this and explain the form of treatment.

If you are a nonmedical spouse of a doctor, you may prefer seeing a nonmedical therapist because you will not have to worry about dual doctor alignment, that is, that your physician spouse and the treating physician will collude in a two-against-one dynamic. This is a very realistic fear and is best discussed ahead of time directly with your physician therapist, should you choose one. One of the reasons why a dual doctor alignment can occur, and quite unconsciously at that, is because the commonality in personality, training, and experience of many doctors does not allow objectivity to occur in the sessions. Another reason is that in many communities, physicians know or know of each other through professional channels not open to nonmedical spouses. This medical networking allows doctors to meet each other and cultivate the referral process. It is also how doctors weigh the many factors involved in deciding who they let treat them when they are in need of medical care. Therefore, when your husband or wife calls Dr. X to ask for marital therapy, they may have already met or have heard of each other. When the two of you arrive for the initial visit with Dr. X, you may feel "one down" or not quite on equal ground.

PSYCHIATRISTS

Because psychiatrists are medically trained, they are in the best position to offer you a thorough biopsychosocial assessment of your marital situation and to implement broad-based treatment. This is especially important if you are symptomatic (e.g., depressed, anxious, phobic, or somatizing). A psychiatrist should be able to determine if you are clinically ill (as a result of marital difficulty, as a cause of marital difficulty, or completely unrelated to those difficulties) and whether you require individual treatment in addition to, or instead of, marital therapy. Medication may or may not be indicated.

If you have a preexisting medical problem—for example, hypertension, diabetes, coronary artery disease, or thyroid disease—a psychiatrist will have an understanding of the psychological sequelae and concomitants of such disorders. He or she will also know when or if your medication is affecting your mood or your sexual functioning, both of which relate to marital communication. Suspiciousness of one's spouse, including accusations of infidelity, are presenting problems in some marriages, especially in the elderly. A psychiatrist taking a careful history and doing a thorough mental status examination can rule out major psychiatric illness, depression, paranoid disorder, alcoholism, other drug-induced illness or dementia, for instance, when this is the cause.

You may wish to see a psychiatrist because you feel a psychiatrist will appreciate the stresses of medical school, residency training, and the practice of medicine. This feeling may be even more pronounced if many of your difficulties are directly related to your work, or your spouse has concerns related to your work (examples include academic problems, financial indebtedness, conflicts with authority figures, working long hours, and balancing career and family life). Conversely, some doctors feel the opposite and don't wish to see a psychiatrist. Some feel embarrassed about talking with a medical person about their marital concerns; others fear that a psychiatrist will sit in judgment on problems that they perceive as shortcomings. Some doctors fear breaches in confidentiality, that the psychiatrist will discuss "their case" with colleagues and friends they have in common.

I am struck by how often I hear the following or a variation thereof in my practice: "I know that you're friendly with many people that I know. Please don't tell them that we're seeing you, or if you do, please don't tell them any details." At one time I would feel inwardly surprised, hurt, or defensive that physician patients would question or doubt my ethics about matters of privacy and confidentiality. I now realize that when a doctor goes to a psychiatrist with marital troubles there are many possible reasons for such anxiety: he or she already feels embarrassed or ashamed about the predicament and may fear becoming or already being the object of curiosity and gossip in medical circles; doctors are accustomed to discussing patients quite openly with each other and not always with complete appropriateness, sensitivity, and the proper safeguarding of patients' rights to secrecy whatever the medical condition (i.e., there is a precedent for their fears); and many doctors who are friendly with psychiatrists have heard them tell anonymous and titillating anecdotes from their practices in social settings—these physicians do not wish to be included in their psychiatrist's repertoire of stories. I have also heard this from my married medical student patients who find that many residents, whether in psychiatry or not, talk far too openly about their patients' personal problems. What I am getting at is that anxiety about trust is quite understandable, and reassurance about secrecy is absolutely fundamental.

Now having said all of that, in many centers it is not easy to find a psychiatrist who is subspecialized in marital therapy or who even does marital therapy. Many are trained in and prefer to work with individual patients. Those psychiatrists who are trained in family therapy are more apt to be subspecialized in child psychiatry and offer a wide range of therapeutic services to all members of the family, not limiting their practice to marital work for the parents. Even if you consult a psychiatrist for a marital problem, you may then be referred on to a nonmedical therapist for marital help. Sometimes this is because you are a physician patient—not all doctors like treating other doctors. Some admit that they don't feel confident treating other doctors; others generalize about doctor patients. They conclude that they demand too much time and attention, that they have an air of entitlement, that they complain a lot, and that they are intimidating. The sad reality is that many doctors with severe marital difficulties who are quite symptomatic go untreated. One psychiatrist patient of mine told me that he felt like a leper trying to obtain marital help from psychiatrists in our community. "Once I told them over the phone that I was a psychiatrist myself, they suddenly backpedaled, told me apologetically that they were very busy, and gave me the name of one of their colleagues to try."

There are lots of thoughts and questions that run through doctors' minds when they consider seeing a psychiatrist in their community for marital difficulties. I want to conclude this section by mentioning a few of these, because they are common and you may find yourself asking the same ones. "Do I know all the psychiatrists in town? Or all the good ones, anyway?" "How well do I know Dr. X and Dr. Y? Could I tell my troubles to him or her?" "I wonder if I should try to find a psychiatrist who is a complete stranger, rather than someone I've at least met or seen before? But I hate to risk maybe getting a loser and wasting my time." "I wonder what Dr. X's own marriage is like? Traditional? Dual career? Any kids?" "I heard Dr. X is divorced. I wonder if that makes her a better marital therapist? At least she's experienced some marital trouble herself." "I met Dr. B once at a party. He seems a bit uptight and straight to me, but my wife liked him. On the other hand, I find Dr. A too far out for my liking. I don't think he'd be able to empathize with our marital situation at all." "I've been referring patients to Dr. Z for years. I wonder if he would see my husband and me. Now I have to get up the nerve to ask him." "I'll die if he pauses over the phone, or says no. It's taken me so long to come to this decision and to make this call."

SHOULD WE SEE A MALE OR FEMALE THERAPIST?

For many of you this question is largely irrelevant—it does not matter whether your therapist is a man or a woman. Upon further reflection, however, some of you might find that you actually have a preference, or at least some ideas or expectations of a male or female therapist. A minority of doctors and/or their spouses are very clear. They would never see a man, or never see a woman. This singularity of preference may be based on personal psychodynamics plus previous experience with a male or female therapist that was ineffective, negative, or destructive.

Gender is one of the variables that you should keep in mind when selecting a therapist, because it is not insignificant.[7] The other variables are gender free—for instance, type and duration of training in marital therapy, amount of experience in working with couples, and personality. If the therapist you are considering comes highly recommended by a number of other people, is well trained, and is experienced in working with couples, especially medical couples, then his or her gender is less important. There are exceptions, though. Some therapists work well with male doctors whose marriages are on the traditional end of the spectrum, but these same therapists do not fare as well with dual career marriages, especially women doctors' marriages. For other therapists, the converse is true.

The breadth and duration of clinical know-how is so important because a good marital therapist must be able to perceive and be sensitive to *both* the female experience and the male experience in marriage. As a patient in marital therapy, you can sense immediately, or certainly after a few visits, if you or your spouse is not being understood and respected for your differing feelings, attitudes, and behaviors toward each other. Any sense of the therapist's siding with you or your spouse because of his or her gender should be noted and aired. Your therapist should be able to respond to your query in a nondefensive manner, welcoming your observation of gender issues in marital therapy as a significant matter for discussion.

Your wishes about the gender of the therapist may be different from your spouse's, and this may pose a problem if a compromise can't be reached. I have had some interesting examples of this in my practice. A number of doctors' wives, some of them doctors themselves, have told me that their preference was to see a woman marital therapist (for a variety of reasons), but they capitulated to their husbands' wishes to see a man. Most often their physician husbands are quite sexist (I don't mean this pejoratively; I am being clinical and rather dispassionate) and do not respect women professionals as equal to men. Some of them taunt and provoke women professionals in such an aggressive and insulting manner that even I as a man feel defensive and angered. Their marital problems get played out in my office, and this dynamic can then be directly addressed. I also get an opportunity to reach behind their sexist persona, so to speak, to enable them to come in touch with their insecurities and feelings of inferiority toward women, especially strong and capable women in authority. When these feelings are addressed, these doctors and their wives feel a lot better about this particular gender dynamic. Some of these men have also stated that they feared that a woman therapist would automatically side with their wives, because they have a lifelong history of upsetting and alienating women with their chauvinistic, abrasive style.

The scholarly research on changing gender roles, mostly by women theorists and clinicians, since the resurgence of the women's movement in the late 1960s has been phenomenal. Never before has there been such intensive study of the changing roles of women and men in our society, both in the workplace and in marriage and families. Much of this research is being incorporated into the curricula of training programs for marital and family therapy, but there is a long way to go. Therapists themselves must not only keep abreast of this research but also incorporate it into their daily work with couples. Examples of clinical situations with gender-related underpinnings include physically and sexually abused wives, custody battles, battering husbands, alcoholic wives, workaholic husbands, depressed homemakers, women and men suffering role strain, abandoned wives, and child support payments that are unmet—and these happen in many doctors' marriages. The more skill that your therapist has with these problems, the easier it will be for all of you to work together toward solving your marital difficulties.

HOW CAN WE TELL IF THE THERAPY IS HELPING?

"How can we tell if the therapy is helping?" The answer to this question is simple. There should be some feeling of change, however small, after four to six visits, or even earlier depending upon the magnitude and duration of your conflict. What do I mean by change? You should feel a bit better, less symptomatic, less angry, less anxious, less sad, or more hopeful. Your spouse should feel better, too, though not necessarily simultaneously or in the same way that you feel. Marital therapy visits vary in their intensity and their impact—some visits will feel more productive than others and you will feel buoyant; other visits feel less meaningful or are lackluster and you will wonder if you're getting anywhere.

What are other signs of change? Your communication with each other should be easier. This may mean that you return to communicating well ("like we used to"), or you begin to communicate as you never have before. You should now be able to discuss more delicate subjects, you disclose more, you listen better, you learn new things about each other, you set aside more time together for talking, and that time feels well spent. If your dialogue was highly intellectualized, stiff, and mechanical, the trend now should be toward more intimate and emotionally connected speech. Conversely, if your dialogue had been of a high intensity with a lot of emotion and volatility, you should now be moving toward a calmer and more relaxed exchange with one another. If your communication before was highly defensive and hostile, you should now be beginning to feel more trusting, less vulnerable, less attacked, and less attacking of your spouse.

Issues and decisions should be clearer. There should be fewer misunderstandings, less second-guessing of your spouse, and a greater sense of predictability and knowing where you stand with each other. You and your spouse should feel less ambivalent about the concerns in your relationship and less ambivalent about each other. If your marriage has been in quite serious trouble, and if you or your spouse has been wrestling with whether to remain together, a decision one way or the other should be easier after a few visits with your marital therapist. It is very common to feel hopeless about your marriage when you begin marital therapy. The feeling is, "I can't live like this any longer; unless something changes, I want to leave." For most couples, things do change; there is a glimmer of hope and the urgent need to separate passes. For other couples, things can't change; this is what becomes clear after a few visits with your marital therapist. There may be a sense of relief in this discovery: You have come to a decision to separate, finally, after months or years of agonizing.

It is imperative that you have a frank discussion with your therapist if, after a few visits, you feel there is no change or a worsening of the situation. You should have this discussion even if only one of you feels this way. It is important to have this feeling validated and clarified. The feeling of "no change" may be part of a problem with your expectations; that is, you are expecting change too soon given the duration of your problems and the number of appointments, or you are expecting major change when only minor change is possible. If this is the case, your therapist should be able to explore these expectations with you in an open and respectful manner so that you feel understood and also relieved that you are not wasting your time. You should end up feeling comfortable about continuing in therapy—not coerced, bullied, or shamed into continuing.

If after a few visits you feel that things are "worsening," your therapist should want to know what you mean by this. Do you mean that you and your spouse are fighting more? Or are further estranged? Or more unhappy together? Or do your children seem affected now? Does a worsening situation mean that one of you seems fine but the other is more symptomatic—anxious, depressed, hostile, cold, drinking, or avoidant? Paradoxically, your sense of things worsening could mean that things are getting better and that the therapy is working! Deeply buried issues are now being aired and discussed. But once again, if this is the case, your therapist should be able to explain to you in a comforting and reassuring manner that some couples feel worse before they feel better. Further, this phenomenon should fluctuate from day to day, or week to week. This feeling of worsening should not continue unabated without good periods interspersed. Your therapist should monitor these feelings carefully at each visit, because your concern about them should become his or her concern as well. Acknowledging this situation, your therapist may suggest a change in format, perhaps a change in frequency of appointments, or perhaps a second opinion.

What do you do if your attempts and efforts to discuss any of these concerns with your therapist are thwarted or dismissed? What should you do if you receive an angry or defensive response from your therapist? What if your therapist blames you (e.g., "Well, you're not working very hard"), and you feel that you're doing your best? What if you didn't feel comfortable with your therapist at the beginning and after several visits feel the same way? What if everyone you know likes your therapist and he or she comes highly recommended, but you just don't feel right? What if you just don't trust or respect the person? The answer is obvious. Go elsewhere!

A feeling that your therapist is not being neutral and is siding more with your spouse than yourself is not uncommon in marital therapy. Feeling that your therapist is siding more with you than your spouse is less common. Although there are many factors, both conscious and unconscious, that contribute to this phenomenon, there are two major sets of variables—yours and the therapist's. You must discuss this feeling with your therapist, and further, you should feel welcomed in mentioning a need to come to an understanding about it. This is a trust issue that must be clarified; therapy cannot proceed without it. Seasoned and well-trained therapists will not feel attacked or defensive about your bringing up this observation and feeling. On the contrary, they will want to know more about it, they will want you to express all of your additional feelings about it (i.e., including possible feelings of alienation, anger, being ganged up on, rejection, and disappointment in therapy), and they will openly examine their own feelings about and behavior toward you and your spouse in the session. Therapist responses might include the following: "I agree with you 100%. In fact, I was going to bring this up today myself. I have found myself siding with your wife in her frustration with your continued drinking. You must feel picked on." Or, "I wasn't aware of siding with your wife, but as I listen to you describe my actions and quote what I've been saying the past couple of visits, I see what you mean. I'll certainly think about this some more and watch it." Or, "I'm pretty sure I'm not siding with your wife, but

I'm glad you brought it up and that you've talked about your feelings here. It's essential that you feel comfortable with me and can trust me. Let's see how it goes for the next session or two and discuss it again."

Each of you should have a feeling that your therapist has your best interests at heart and is there to be supportive and to assist while you negotiate your way clear of problems. You are paying for a professional service and therefore have a right to expect certain things of a therapist. Once again, I urge you to discuss openly those expectations of therapy that you feel are not being realized and changes that you find are not happening. Although most people approach marital therapy with quite realistic intentions ("I know you're not a miracle worker"; "I'm not expecting you to wave a magic wand"), it is impossible to know how much change might be achieved. You can't help feeling disappointed when change is slow, minimal, painful, or heading in a frightening direction, for instance, separation. By talking about these issues with your therapist you should be able to answer the questions that arise from your disappointment: Are our expectations too high? Are we working hard enough in therapy? Is it common to feel this let down, and if so, are there any other reasons for it? Is this therapist not for us, and should we go elsewhere?

WHY IS MY SPOUSE SO RESISTANT TO MARITAL THERAPY?

I have included a section on spouses' resistance to marital therapy because it is very common, not just in doctors and their spouses, but in married couples in general. Many individuals go to their family doctors or to a psychiatrist (or other psychotherapist) with a vague complaint of uneasiness or unhappiness that is, in essence, a marital problem. They cannot get their spouse to come in with them for marital therapy with or without their doctor's assistance. In other homes, the marital problem is obvious, undisputed, and openly acknowledged by both partners, yet one of them adamantly refuses to seek help. Eventually some of these spouses will go for marital help, but not until separation is seriously threatened, is imminent, or has occurred.

Why is this? What are some of the reasons for resistance to marital treatment? There are many reasons, some of which are general, and some of which are specific to doctors alone. By mentioning these factors I hope to shed light on and add to your understanding of the so-called reluctant spouse, who is frequently labeled as selfish, uncaring, lazy, or unmotivated. This is not to say that husbands and wives don't fit these descriptions—indeed, some do, at least in part—but in my experience they are in the minority.

PRIVATE INDIVIDUAL

Some people are simply private. Their needs for privacy vary—from a little to a lot. These individuals do not talk easily with anyone, including their spouses. In fact, many of my patients warn me to go easy, or not to expect much self-disclosure when, or if, I am given the opportunity to interview their spouse. "My husband doesn't discuss anything personal with anyone, except me, and only occasionally at that, if I really work at it" is a typical statement.

This privacy can mean many different things. Usually it is a life-long trait that dates back to childhood. There may be genetic and familial factors, including paranoid traits in the person or in the family. Some of it may be based in shyness, or feelings of unworthiness, or poor self-esteem. There may be a history of betrayal of privacy over the years, hence a need to not say much based in mistrust of others. Some private individuals have never felt anyone was interested in what they had to say, or they have been ridiculed or demeaned in the past, so they say nothing.

SELF-RELIANCE

Many people are accustomed to resolving problems on their own and have always functioned in this way. Usually this has served them well, and they take pride in their self-sufficiency and independence. In my work as a psychiatrist, I marvel at the number of people I see in a year who give histories of unhappy childhoods, major personal losses, and other stressful periods in their lives for which they received no outside help. Further, they have often struggled through periods in their lives successfully and courageously without talking to anyone. Various coping strategies have worked for them, including a "nose to the grindstone" approach to life, rugged determination to survive, focused thought, contemplation, hope, prayer, and so forth.

Unfortunately, these same skills, based in individualism, do not work as well with marital stress. They are effective in recognizing and understanding the issues, but not in overcoming them. I am talking about dialogue and discussion here as a fundamental exercise in solving marital differences and unhappiness. It is precisely this shared communication that is missing and longed for by people who are married to these resolute women and men, who demean marital therapy as a waste of their time and the therapist's time. These individualists tend to compare past stresses with their marital stress in an attempt to gauge by magnitude alone the necessity of, or their worthiness for, professional help. This was exemplified by one of my patients, the only member of his family to survive the Holocaust, whose opening words to me were, "I'm embarrassed to be sitting here with a marriage problem given what I've been through in my life."

Self-reliance in doctors is classic and seems to be multidetermined. People with this trait are attracted to medicine and, once accepted into medical school, do well if they can maintain it and "not rock the boat." The process of medical education itself rewards self-reliance and denial of one's own needs and human vulnerabilities. The mandate is to work hard, to excel, and to serve others. This process is further reinforced by residency training and the practice of medicine (or its equivalents— teaching, research, administration, etc.) after that. Our patients and students expect us to be self-reliant, and we expect it in ourselves. In my work with doctors I am used to seeing many women and men who feel terribly frustrated and annoyed at themselves for having to come for marital assistance.

NEGATIVE PREVIOUS TREATMENT

Having had an earlier experience with a therapist that was not helpful, or worse, destructive, is a major deterrent to embracing professional help again. Although this experience might have occurred some time in the distant past, the negative memory may be very strong, with far-reaching consequences. Even if the person does agree to try some form of help again, it will not be easy to get beyond the feelings of wariness, mistrust, and lack of enthusiasm. There may be resultant negativity toward all mental health professionals, or only specific disciplines within the profession (e.g., psychiatrists but not psychologists), or specific sexes (e.g., men but not women). The previous negative treatment experience might have been as an individual or a couple, in this marriage or in a former relationship or marriage.

Let me give some verbatim examples of what I mean: "I saw a psychiatrist for several months when I was a teenager, but he never said a word to me—I suppose that was part of his technique—but I never thought he was quite real." "I got depressed in second-year medical school, but I think my shrink had more problems than me. I had a lot of sexual problems at the time, and every time I began to discuss them his facial twitch worsened, or he blushed. I decided to just get better on my own." "When I was a fourth-year medical student my father died. I got fairly depressed but not clinically so, if you know what I mean—no sleep change, no weight loss, not suicidal or anything. I sought out a psychiatrist because I wanted to talk about my dad and our relationship, which was very complicated. My doctor insisted that I take antidepressants; when I told him that I wanted and needed psychotherapy he accused me of being a smart-ass and then lectured me about medical students thinking they know all about psychiatry after a six-week clerkship! I never went back." "I started in psychotherapy with Dr. X during my residency, and at first it went very well. After several months, though, he began to talk more and more about himself and how unhappily married he was. I felt sorry for him. He called me once at home, and he sounded drunk. In our next session I urged him to get help himself. He turned on me in quite an accusatory way. I backed off and was afraid of him from then on." "My first wife and I saw a marriage therapist together. Although I was pretty immature in those days, I just ran circles around her. We went for months and learned nothing." "My husband and I saw Dr. Y two years ago when we were in crisis. What disturbed me was that I always felt one down in the sessions. I really felt like I was the nagging doctor's wife and they, the two of them, were my doctors!"

These examples of previous therapy experiences may sound beyond belief to some of you and all too real to others of you. But these perceptions and the memories of some people who have sought professional help in the past will greatly influence their decision to ever seek help again or color their approach to treatment if they do seek it. Any of you with spouses resistant to marital therapy would be wise to explore their earlier therapy experiences with them.

SEX OF YOUR SPOUSE

As a general rule, men are more resistant to marital therapy than women. Much of this is based in what I have described already: a need for privacy ("I'm not telling my marital troubles to the world"); a tendency toward self-reliance ("What can a therapist do? We can solve these problems ourselves"); or a previous therapy experience that was negative ("I've been that route before; those people are useless"). Reaching out for professional help also runs against the grain of the traditional male sex role; some men feel that it is a sign of weakness or less than masculine to be in therapy. Still other men feel suspect at the whole notion of marital therapy, which has as its basic premise and emphasis open communication and disclosure of feelings. This may feel awkward and foreign to them, and also intimidating, because their wives are more experienced, knowledgeable, and adept at this type of exercise.

FAMILY HISTORY OF PSYCHIATRIC ILLNESS

Anyone in medicine who has psychiatric illness, especially severe or major psychiatric illness, in his or her family cannot help but be affected in many different ways. If it is in first-degree relatives such as parents or siblings, you have felt the psychological effects of living with someone who is, was, or has been ill from time to time. You may worry about genetic transmission. You will be affected by the stigma of psychiatric illness in our society.[8] Your attitudes toward psychiatrists will be colored by the care that someone close to you has received. All of this can contribute to ambivalence you may feel about marital therapy. Will my therapist focus on me more than my spouse? Will the therapist blame me for the bulk of the marital distress? Will the therapist "label" me because of psychiatric illness in my family? Will I have to take medication?

MISCELLANEOUS CONCERNS

Say you are a doctor with marital troubles and feel fine about seeing a psychiatrist. If your spouse is nonmedical, he or she may fear that you'll align with the psychiatrist, or the psychiatrist with you, because you have medicine in common. Even if you are in different specialties, there is a commonality of language, custom, and purpose from which laypersons, including spouses, can feel excluded. This may be even worse if you and the doctor are both of the same sex, because dual doctor alignment is compounded by concerns about dual gender alignment. If you have had therapy some other time in your life and it went well, your positive feelings about the whole process may contrast quite starkly with your spouse's reservations about marital treatment. If you are not very empathic and underestimate your spouse's anxiety, you will not be very successful in reassuring him or her. You may have forgotten your own anxieties the first time you sought therapy.

Say you are not a doctor, but your husband or wife is. You feel fine about seeing a psychiatrist or therapist of any discipline. Your spouse may have reservations for all of the reasons I have mentioned earlier, including denial that there is any problem in the first place. There may be a feeling of embarrassment and failure, coupled with a tendency to minimize the distress. You sense that your spouse is putting his or her patients ahead of you in importance and doesn't have time for marital therapy. You back off for a while, but if there is no change, you bring it up again. Eventually you may have to resort to separation to get your message across.

One final concern. You and your spouse's cultural, racial, ethnic, and religious backgrounds strongly influence attitudes toward marital therapy. The idea of recognizing and noting marital disharmony and then speaking to a therapist may be anathema to a member of one culture, only to be eagerly pursued by a member of another culture. If your backgrounds are the same or quite similar, and you agree to seek marital help, you may have a shared problem—finding a therapist who has something in common with the two of you or at least an empathic understanding of your lives and how they've been shaped. If the two of you have had very different backgrounds, and this is common in medicine, you may have difficulty finding a therapist you both trust and one you feel on an equal footing with. It is quite understandable for your spouse to feel reserved about treatment if the therapist you have in mind is of the same race or religion or country of origin as you are, but one that is different from his or her own. This reticence will be increased if you already know the therapist through professional channels, or if you have already begun individual therapy with him or her. International medical graduates living in North America feel this exquisitely; sometimes their American-born spouses underestimate the magnitude of their feelings. I cannot emphasize these feelings enough as factors that make people resistant to marital therapy.

WHAT KINDS OF MARITAL THERAPY ARE THERE?

Marital therapy can be classified in various ways, but for my purposes here I want to mention only two: typology according to theorctical orientation, and typology according to format.[9] With regard to the former, there are three commonly described theoretical approaches: behavioral, systems, and psychoanalytic-psychodynamic.

A *behavioral approach* is grounded in learning theory, wherein your therapist helps you identify the unsuccessful ways you and your spouse interact and teaches the two of you new ways of interacting. For example, you are chronically annoyed that your husband doesn't put his dirty dishes in the dishwasher after snacking. He is chronically annoyed that you keep him waiting when the two of you are going out for the evening. Your therapist will assist each of you to work toward changing your own behavior over an agreed-upon time period, say two weeks. Your therapist will also assist each of you in negotiating a concrete and specifically enjoyed reward for a change of behavior. As an example: You may agree to bake your husband his favorite pie; he may agree to take you out to your favorite restaurant for dinner.

A *systems theory approach* to marital conflicts presumes that a change in one family member brings about a change somewhere else in the family system. For example, your daughter has anorexia nervosa, and it is a worry to you and your spouse. She receives individual treatment and begins to improve. Unless you and your spouse are part of this treatment, family systems theory argues that one of you or some other family member may now become symptomatic with a new problem.

The *psychoanalytic-psychodynamic perspective* has inner, intrapsychic factors, conscious and unconscious, that affect many things in marriage, including whom we marry and how we interact with our spouses. For example, many men who recoil at their wives' yelling at their children are reacting to and reliving their own mothers' yelling at them as children. Many adults who are panic-stricken that their husband or wife will abandon them suffer from separation anxiety rooted in their own childhood. Perhaps they feared their parents would separate, or perhaps the parents actually did separate.

Miscellaneous theoretical backgrounds that may influence your therapist's approach include communication theory and transactional analysis, Gestalt theory and "here-and-now" techniques, dream analysis and dream work in therapy, role-playing, and feminist theory, which espouses egalitarian principles in marriage as a challenge to the unhealthy values and expectancies of traditional forms of marriage. Many therapists use an eclectic approach that is an amalgam of these various theories and schools of thought in their clinical work.

Let us return now to the second way of classifying marital therapy, that is, according to format. The most common approach is conjoint therapy, wherein both of you are seen together at the same time by the same therapist. Some therapists are quite rigid about this. They are not interested in seeing either of you alone and adamantly refuse to do so. Nor will they speak to you alone over the phone. Their philosophy is that they do not want to know anything that the two of you have not shared and discussed with each other. Most therapists are not this rigid; they use a conjoint format but usually have one, perhaps two, sessions with each of you alone to learn about your personal and family backgrounds.

The next most commonly used format is concurrent marital therapy, wherein each of you is in individual treatment with the same therapist. Some therapists combine the concurrent and conjoint approaches. Other therapists practice collaborative therapy—in this format, each of you would be undergoing individual therapy with different therapists who are in regular contact with each other with your consent. Some therapists, usually of the opposite sex, work together as cotherapists, that is, they see you and your spouse together for conjoint therapy. And finally, some therapists, solely or as cotherapists, run couples' groups comprised of from three to five couples meeting regularly for group therapy.

Although marital therapy for many couples is relatively brief, six to twelve hourly visits at weekly to biweekly intervals, your situation may not lend itself to any conventionally prescribed or predictable approach. This is not necessarily an ominous prognostic statement, nor is it necessarily a statement of severe marital or personal unhappiness. Some couples need a longer period of time to settle in with their therapist; this includes getting to underlying issues, especially sexual concerns, which are harder to talk about. Some couples need longer time intervals of, say, three to four weeks between visits, perhaps because the visits are emotionally upsetting, perhaps to have more time to work on things at home. Some couples need to experiment with different formats at different times with their therapist in order to uncover certain personal and interpersonal problems and to begin to tackle them.

What do you do if your therapist recommends individual treatment for each of you? This might occur after an initial conjoint consultation visit if, at that point, your therapist feels it is not possible to work with the two of you together. Find out his or her reasons for this decision. Is there too much tension or hostility between the two of you to begin to work at communication improvement? Is there a motivation discrepancy? Is one of you motivated to work while the other isn't? Would conjoint work be counterproductive, inefficient, or perhaps inappropriate and destructive to the marriage at this point? It is important to have a sufficient and convincing explanation from your therapist so that you can trust and respect his or her counsel. I know several couples who were told after one visit that conjoint therapy wasn't right for them. No reasons were given. They felt lost, disappointed, rejected, unworthy, and frightened that their marriage was hopeless and separation inevitable. Further, some felt quite intimidated by the suggestion of individual therapy, if it was even mentioned. What they heard from their therapist (upon reading between the lines) was, "Your marriage is a mess. You're both screwed up. Each of you needs treatment."

Sometimes individual treatment is suggested down the road a bit. Conjoint therapy has worked, but only to a point. Both you and your therapist may feel stuck, as if nothing is happening. Issues and themes in the visits feel repetitive. At this point, you may not be against individual therapy; indeed, you may welcome it, especially if your therapist prefers to continue seeing you. Being referred to a new therapist is another matter; once again, be sure to ask your therapist as many questions as you need to, in order to make the transition as easy as possible.

A more complicated matter arises when or if your marital therapist suggests individual treatment for only one of you. Unless you have already come to this conclusion yourself and actually feel quite accepting of this change, if not excited about it, then this kind of suggestion can be extremely upsetting. It is normal to feel a range of things—defensive, angry, hurt, singled out, blamed, "sick"—you name it. Your reaction will be tempered by your therapist's manner and how sensitively he or she explains the reasons behind the suggestion. If you feel that your spouse needs and/or could benefit from individual therapy too (as opposed to a purely tit-for-tat feeling), you must say so. Only in this way can you learn your therapist's reasons for not suggesting this individual treatment already, as well as your spouse's reaction to your statement. Dialogue and discussion might ensue, at the end of which your spouse and therapist might decide to do some work together as well.

I cannot emphasize enough the importance of your having a clear explanation from your therapist about the reasons for and anticipated benefits of individual treatment. Without this explanation, it will not be possible for you to work with your therapist, or a new therapist, in a safe and mutually respectful way. Without this rapport, you'll get nowhere. If you're a woman, your marital therapist is a man, and you feel sexism and sexist bias is a factor in his reasons for suggesting individual treatment for you and not your husband, say so. If his response is defensive and he is not open to discussing this very fundamental matter in therapy, get a second opinion from a more enlightened therapist. If you lack the confidence and assertiveness (do not feel badly about this, many people do) to question your therapist on possible sexist factors contaminating his judgment, and if this feeling persists, I think you should get a second opinion. You should not have to feel that intimidated (ideally, not intimidated at all!) by your therapist.

Many couples in conflict feel competitive, touchy, hypersensitive, and vulnerable with each other. When you're unhappy and angry with each other, you also feel demoralized. You search for reasons for your marital deterioration. You do question the mental health of your spouse—and if you're fairly open and mature, you question your own mental health. In fights, you may be accused of being "crazy," "screwed up," "neurotic," "a drunk," "frigid," and so forth. You may have accused your spouse of all of these things yourself or perhaps used a different litany of condemnations. Therefore, to be asked by your therapist to consider individual therapy is jarring, frightening, and "confirms" your innermost doubts about your mental health.

In general, marital therapy calls for a more active and directive role on the part of the therapist than does individual therapy. There should be a comfortable balance established so that you and your spouse have an opportunity to express your ideas and feelings on a shared conflict as well as receive assistance in doing so. You should feel that your therapist is actively engaged in your work together, and after the individual introductory visits is offering some observations and commentary. If this is not happening, address it at the time or in the next session. You are entitled to an explanation and an invitation to discuss this situation further. Your therapist may conclude that it's premature to give feedback, or that in his or her mind it has been happening all along. Ask for elaboration. Ask for the rationale behind his or her particular style. Only in this way can you become clearer about expectations (yours and your therapist's) and whether or not you are with the right therapist.

It is best to think of your marital therapist as a trained professional who can help you in at least two ways—as a consultant and as an assistant. Although the process begins with a consultation, these functions do not necessarily follow each other but proceed simultaneously— your therapist will be assessing your marriage on an ongoing basis while assisting the two of you from session to session. You can expect your therapist to determine the conflict areas and your individual contributions to these conflicts. By making these underlying dynamics more obvious and visible to the two of you, your therapist aids in increasing your understanding. He or she can then help as you both work toward eliminating habitual and ineffective communication and adopting new ways. Your therapist provides a facilitating and encouraging environment in which to begin this work, and to continue it with you, as you go about your daily lives.

You are most likely to become disappointed in your therapist if you defer too much to his or her authority or if your therapist assumes too much authority, power, and control. You must be prepared to work, individually and together, even if the work feels highly experimental. All marriages are unique. At heart, only you and your spouse really know what is best for the two of you. Your therapist should not make you feel that there is only one way, the therapist's way, to live your marriage. On the contrary, you should sense a flexibility and assurance in your therapist as you explore new and exciting ideas and emotions with one another. Your therapist's training and experience with other couples helps to light the way, but should never dictate it. That is not therapy.

Regardless of their theoretical orientation to marital discord and treatment, most therapists will focus on the current issues and problems in your marriage that are causing the distress. With some of you, though, this is not enough. It will be necessary to make connections between present behavior, values, and attitudes and the past—in childhood, in one's parents' marriage, or in a previous marriage or committed relationship. This is not just an intellectual exercise but a means of your reaching a better and more sensible understanding of why you act and react the way that you do with your spouse in particular circumstances. Only with this emotional knowledge can you begin to work at change; and if change is not possible, at least you and your spouse can work toward acceptance of the situation, if that is possible.

Dr. and Mrs. Q came to see me at Mrs. Q's request. Her concern was that she and her husband had become so busy in their daily lives that it was beginning to affect their solidarity as a couple. She felt that they bickered more with each other, that they were socializing less and less together, and that her husband was becoming "sexually peculiar." What she meant by this (and Dr. Q agreed) was that more and more he was disinterested in sex and, further, didn't want to be touched in any sort of erotic way. This had not been a problem earlier in their relationship. Dr. Q had always been very interested in sex and was relaxed about it. In fact, it was Mrs. Q who had evolved into a more sexually interested and confident woman after many years of shyness and sexual awkwardness. Both Dr. Q and Mrs. Q noted that his sexual "uptightness" was worse if she had had anything to drink; she needn't be intoxicated, which she seldom was anyway—one drink would put him off.

I arranged individual visits with each of them. During my session with Dr. Q, I learned that his mother had died eighteen months earlier. He told me that he was puzzled by his reaction to her death. What he meant was that he found himself greatly preoccupied with her, not only in his working life, but in his dreams. He had experienced many emotions typical of bereavement but felt that his preoccupation was abnormal in duration and in intensity. I found myself agreeing, because he spent virtually the rest of his hour with me talking about her. At times, he was excited and animated as he described her many talents and achievements; at other times, he was swept away with sorrow and rage as he described her courageous fight with cancer. I decided to postpone conjoint work until I had a more complete understanding of Dr. Q through more individual sessions. Both Dr. Q and Mrs. Q consented to this plan.

These individual visits were enlightening and helped to explain Dr. Q's change in sexual desire and comfort. He was an only child who from the age of six was raised by his mother alone after his father's death. Dr. Q stated that during his adolescence his mother "went a little strange." She drank a lot for several months after the man she was about to marry left her for another woman. Late at night on a couple of occasions, she crawled into bed with her son "just to be comforted, I guess." Once she was naked. Dr. Q recalled many upsetting memories of his mother from this period, memories that made him feel angry, but also very ashamed and sad. "It was all very subtle. Mother would make comments on my body when I left for school or when I was going out—that I was becoming a man, wondering if girls found me sexy. At other times, she'd ask me if she looked sexy. The hardest time for me was when she had been drinking and I came in from being out for the evening. She was always up, in her dressing gown, with this look and manner which was, well, seductive. I was so uptight, I was afraid to go near her—and the perfume—I've never told anyone about this. For years I thought I was just imagining things. It's only been since medical school, as I learned more about incest in families, that I wondered about my relationship with my mother and how I feel about women in general and about sex."

What this example illustrates is not only how the past affects the present but how important it is to be able to make the necessary connections in order to change. Dr. Q found himself feeling a lot better after only a few individual therapy sessions. Coming in touch with and discharging many suppressed and repressed feelings about his mother helped him to resolve his bereavement. Understanding how his identity and autonomy as a man felt, to use his word, "invaded" by his mother enabled him to appreciate his sexual wariness and rigidity in the latter months of his marriage. With these insights he was able to work with his wife on many aspects of their relationship. Their verbal and sexual communication improved markedly after only three or four conjoint sessions.

WHAT HAPPENS IN MARITAL THERAPY?

By describing briefly how I approach a couple with a marital problem, I hope to allay some of the anxiety that is omnipresent in people coming to see a marital therapist. I want also to try to simplify what marital therapy is all about.

During the first interview I try to determine the surface complaints that the couple brings to treatment. I also try to understand each partner's sense of the problem areas and whether they are in agreement. I want to know how long they have felt symptomatic and whether they have some thoughts about possible contributing factors to the surface complaints. I learn whether any previous marital therapy has been obtained and what each person's feelings were about that treatment.

If there have been previous separations, I want to know about those separations, what the reasons for separating were, and the circumstances that led to their reunion. I try to obtain some sense of the couple's shared interests and also determine what individual and separate interests each member of the couple has. How committed each person is to the marriage is important, as well as their commitment to marital therapy.

If time permits, in the first interview I like to get some background about their relationship. How did they meet? How long was their courtship? Did problems arise during the courtship? Did they live together before the marriage? If so, how was that period? How was their early sexual experience together? Were there any problems? Has there been a change in the sexual pattern, that is, in the frequency and quality of their lovemaking over the course of the marriage? If so, in what ways? Do they feel that any changes in their sexual relationship may be related to other problem areas or external stresses?

After the initial conjoint visit, I like to have at least one, occasionally two, individual visits with each person. These visits equalize the amount of time spent alone with me. Rapport is strengthened, and neither partner feels shortchanged or "one down." Each person is given an opportunity to tell his or her story without the partner contradicting or censoring. I also use these sessions to learn about things from each partner that have not been shared with the spouse and that may be critical to my assessment, treatment approach, and prognosis. Examples of such information are undisclosed previous marriages, previous pregnancies and abortions, previous psychiatric treatment, extramarital sexual activity, incest, and homosexuality.

I use individual visits to obtain selective details about each partner's personal and family histories. I like to have some sense of their ability to cope with their frustrations, to adapt to stress, and to handle disappointment. I also try to get a sense of each partner's level of self-confidence and maturity. How capable is each partner of independence, and what are their respective capacities for love? How able are they to give support and to accept support from each other?

With regard to family history, I like to obtain some information regarding each partner's family. How have they viewed their parents' marriage or marriages? How happily married are or were their parents? Have there been any separations or divorces in their families? How did their parents resolve their differences? Were there arguments, physical violence, or mutual withdrawal? Was the father the sole or principal wage earner? Was the mother at home full-time while the patient was growing up? Did she return to paid work later? Was there strict division of labor in the home based on sex? How were the finances managed? Did the parents spend leisure time together? Is there any family history of alcoholism or psychiatric illness?

With regard to each partner's personal history, I try to determine if there were any developmental problems during childhood and adolescence. When did dating begin? Were there any problems involved in dating? Were there any serious long-term relationships before marriage? How was the person's first sexual experience? How much sexual experience, if any, did they have before meeting each other? Were there problems with this? Have there been any previous marriages? If so, when did the marriages occur, and what was the duration of the marriages? Were there children by a previous marriage? What were the reasons for separation and divorce? Was there time between the separation and the present relationship for some resolution and independent living to develop?

This short synopsis gives you some idea of what might happen in your early visits with your marital therapist. Although all therapists work somewhat differently according to their own training, experience, and personal style, most approach and assess couples in much the same way I have described. Because you and your spouse have your own unique backgrounds and highly idiosyncratic way of being with each other, you can see how certain elements of your "story" will be focused upon more than others. This focus is what enriches your marital therapy and moves you onto a different plane with your therapist away from superficial chitchat and advice giving.

WHAT CAN WE EXPECT OF THERAPY?

The object of therapy, of course, is to feel better, even if the route is a bit circuitous. As I have stated earlier, you should feel clearer about yourself, your spouse, and your marriage if therapy is helping. Understandably, this process may be painful at times because embarking on marital therapy means taking a look at things that have made no sense to you, or facing things that you have been frightened by for some time. Many people fear that marital therapy will cause them to separate. In reality, marital therapy can't *make* you separate. Couples who do separate in the course of marital therapy were already on their way before starting; the therapy has merely affirmed the inevitability of separation or the need to separate. The number of people who do separate with marital therapy is actually quite small compared with the number who *fear* separation. Your therapist should be able to help allay this anxiety, both directly by explaining it to you, and indirectly by his or her manner.

You can expect a safe, mutually respectful, and nonjudgmental relationship with your therapist. You and your spouse must both feel this, even if you don't always feel it to the same degree, or at the same time. This type of relationship must be there as the foundation of your therapy. Being nonjudgmental is not the same as being unfeeling, unreactive, passive, or detached. Indeed, at times your therapist may need to be very direct and confrontative. But it is possible to be this way in a firm yet kind and nonmoralistic way.

You should be able to discharge feelings in therapy both about and toward each other. Your therapist may deliberately attempt to mobilize feelings that are an appropriate response to your situation. This "mobilization" is especially critical if these are unconscious feelings or feelings hiding behind certain behaviors that are upsetting to your spouse. Unleashing these feelings enables you to feel better and perhaps less tense and enhances understanding between you and your spouse. For those of you who have no difficulty releasing feelings, or perhaps feel overwhelmed by feeling (especially negative feeling) in your marriage, your therapist will work toward dampening some of this emotion or at least monitoring it. Attention will be directed toward slowing things down and listening to one another. You should not feel that you're spending every session fighting with each other in your therapist's office!

Here's an example of interpreting and mobilizing feeling. Many of you have heard of passive–aggressive behavior—some of you may have been accused of it. Basically it means not being in touch with or openly acknowledging the feeling that should accompany an interaction. Instead of getting angry at your spouse when you feel attacked or ordered to do something, you smile and proceed not to do that task by forgetting it, or procrastinating, or by doing it poorly. Should such an interaction occur in a session with your therapist, wherein he or she perceives that you *should* feel angry in response to something your spouse has said or done, then your therapist may try to get you to talk about your feelings right then—while they are fresh, and in the safety of the office. I say "safety" because these behaviors usually originate in childhood, when to be openly expressive of angry feelings was not tolerated by your parents and may have resulted in punishment or fears of abandonment. When discharging these feelings in the office, you do not experience negative consequences; your fears of punishment or abandonment are allayed.

If it is a serious crisis (e.g., disclosure of an extramarital relationship with possible separation) that brings you to marital therapy, you should be able to count on your therapist until the worst is over and you begin to see your way clearly again. I mean "count on" quite literally—lean on, seek advice from, or take solace from. I say this because in the early days and weeks you are not yourself—you feel regressed, anxious, panicky, confused, indecisive, angry, depressed, out of control, labile, disorganized—and you will not trust your own judgment. Your therapist should understand this and respond with interest and concern. You may also feel quite symptomatic, not sleeping properly, eating poorly, having physical pain, working inefficiently, and so forth. No major life decisions should be made until you begin to feel better and regain your usual level of self-control and purpose.

You may consult a marital therapist about ongoing problems that have been a concern for some time but are not generating a lot of distress in either you or your spouse. In this case, a well-trained and experienced therapist should be able to help the two of you begin to talk again, to communicate more effectively, to make shared decisions more comfortably, and to feel more intimate. Having made the decision to go for marital help together is therapeutic in itself, for it means that each of you is sufficiently concerned about the marriage to want to improve it and preserve it if possible. You are making a commitment to each other to try, and for many people, that is the most they can promise in good faith.

What else can you expect of your therapist? You should be able to gain some perspective on your marriage and the seriousness or non-seriousness of your problems. This perspective is a subtle, largely unspoken, and hard to describe by-product of marital therapy but many people feel it. Young couples especially, or couples who are fairly isolated from their friends and family, may feel quite reassured that their troubles are common, probably temporary, and easily remediable. When the problems are serious, or more serious than originally perceived, your therapist should be committed to assisting as much as possible. No matter how demoralized you feel, and demoralization is very common in couples who go for marital help, you should feel more optimistic about things changing and seeing some light at the end of the tunnel. When demoralization accompanies serious marital conflict and separation is inevitable, you should sense empathic concern from your therapist as well as assistance and support for each of you, and the children, as you proceed.

Finally, you should feel that your therapist is attuned to gender issues in marital therapy. If you and your therapist are of the same sex, you can expect an identification that may be quite straightforward and easily decipherable. However, you should not feel that your therapist colludes with you against your spouse. If this happens inadvertently, your therapist should recognize it and discuss it nondefensively. If you and your therapist are of the opposite sex, you should feel understood, and understood exquisitely. Because your therapist is not of your sex, you should sense that he or she is trying even harder to appreciate your feelings and frustrations in marriage. I cannot emphasize this point too strongly because of the colossal power issues in marriage, and in marital therapy, that are exclusively the province of sex and sex roles.

WHAT IF WE DECIDE TO SEPARATE?

For most couples who separate, the decision has been a long time coming and there has been a lot of discussion for several weeks or months. Often this discussion is conducted without professional help. For others, though, a decision to separate has been made hastily because of a painful marital crisis of some sort, or the decision has not been made jointly. These are the individuals who feel powerless, bereft, abandoned, and discarded. With some marital crises, even the partner who initiates the separation, or the one who leaves, is very ambivalent, unsure, and frightened, although it may appear to the spouse and the outside world that everything is fine with this person. Many of these situations are so calamitous that they can be called psychiatric emergencies.

Why do I say this? Separation is often a response to threat, extreme anxiety, profound depression, and danger. Consequently, as a marital therapist and as a psychiatrist, I have seen people separate under many different and often extreme circumstances: during a manic phase of bipolar affective disorder or in response to a manic spouse; in response to a severely depressed spouse; in the middle of a delirium or in response to a delirious spouse; in response to a paranoid, accusatory, and threatening spouse; in response to a violent and dangerous spouse; in the middle of an alcoholic binge or in response to an incorrigible alcoholic spouse; in the context of an extramarital affair; in the middle of a sexual identity crisis wherein one partner is struggling with homosexual conflicts; during the acute phase of bereavement, especially the death of their child; and in the face of massive and innumerable personal losses. Are we to assume that all of the above separations are due to marital distress in the true sense of the definition? I think not. When or if there is primary marital discord in these situations, it is overshadowed by the larger issue of one or both individuals' psychiatric illness, which is ascendant and requires treatment. Then, and only then, can the marriage be examined.

A psychiatrist can assist in many ways with any of these situations. With your help, he or she should be able to determine the appropriateness and urgency of your desire to separate. Your therapist may suggest that you postpone separation if there is no actual possibility of danger to you or the children, in order to allow more time for complete assessment of each of you and of your marriage. If there is violence and immediate threat of violence, your therapist will support at least a brief, temporary separation in order to create some distance, allow time for cooling off, and facilitate possible attempts at communication later. With each of you feeling less tense, angry, confused, or wounded, it will be easier to try to talk and determine whether it is possible to work toward a reconciliation.

Let us say that your marital situation is not in crisis but has been deteriorating for a long time. You and your spouse do not feel optimistic but consult a marital therapist to see if anything can be done. Or perhaps you and your spouse have already concluded that your marriage is over but call a marital therapist for assistance with separating. These situations are common and legitimate reasons to consult a therapist, who can help a great deal in working with you through the whole separation process. Not only can your therapist make practical suggestions and answer your questions, but it is comforting to have someone available as you and your family negotiate your way through things.

If you have been in marital therapy and separation becomes inevitable, it is important that you don't see separation as a failure of the therapy. You haven't failed, nor has your therapist. There is a lot that your therapist can do to continue to provide help and encouragement. Unfortunately, some therapists feel that their work with a couple ends when or if separation occurs. Even if your therapist suggests names of other therapists for ongoing work, the referral may not be very comforting. You've already established a therapeutic relationship with your therapist, and you probably won't feel like starting over with someone new. If you are in marital therapy with someone or contemplating it, you might want to discuss this matter now or at the outset.

Your feelings when you actually physically separate may come all at once or alternate rapidly. And the feelings range from feeling horrible and lonely to feeling sad and angry to feeling scared stiff to feeling ecstatic. If you have contemplated separation for a long time and have been leading more or less separate lives before physically separating, then you will not find living apart as difficult. Conversely, if you have had virtually no warning about separation and you are opposed to it but have no control over your spouse's desire to separate, the separation will feel terrible.

If your therapist does not do separation therapy, he or she should be able to suggest resources in your community—another therapist for the two of you, or individual therapists for each of you, or a family therapist for all of you if you have children. It will help you to talk to a professional about what to explain to your children about separation, how to tell them, and when to tell them, both in the short term and later. Your therapist may want to meet and talk with your children after they've been told or after you've separated. Depending on their ages, they may welcome a chance to talk to someone who has talked with a lot of children approaching separation. They may have a lot of questions and anxieties that they don't mention to you or your spouse for fear of making things worse or upsetting you more than you are already. Briefly meeting and interviewing your children also enables your therapist to at least have some idea of how they're coping; if there is some concern, then he or she can suggest a more complete assessment and possible treatment by a child psychiatrist. In some communities there are support groups for children going through a family separation, which can be very beneficial. Also, most teachers and school counselors like to know about marital separation in the families of their students so they can watch for any academic or behavioral changes as well as be available for support.

You may want to discuss the pros and cons of divorce mediation with your therapist, as opposed to the more traditional adversarial approach of separate divorce lawyers. You may have questions about joint custody versus solo custody and the implications for the adults and the children, at various ages and stages of their development. Many people who are separating have questions about their common friends and their respective extended families. What are the rules? Are there any? How do I maintain ongoing relationships with these people? Why don't they call me? Are they taking sides?

Like many people approaching marital separation, you may already be involved with someone else. You should discuss this with your therapist because this complicates matters, especially for your children. There will be angry conflicts and hurt feelings around visitation rules and schedules that include the new person. You may have questions about how and when to introduce this person (who is important to you) to your children. Is there an appropriate time? Are they ready? How is this going to affect the ongoing coparenting relationship with your estranged spouse? Your therapist may want to schedule a conjoint visit for you and your estranged spouse to discuss this situation openly and frankly in an attempt to reach some resolution and compromise. If you are not involved with someone else but your spouse is, be certain to be forthright about your feelings regarding your children and the new person. It is normal and common to feel territorial about the children and to feel furious at and/or devastated about your estranged spouse being with someone new. Try to keep your own feelings of hurt and rage toward your spouse separate, if possible, from your children's need and right to see their father or mother. Try not to be punitive by restricting or undermining access and visitation. The adjustment does get easier with passage of time.

What about trial separations? Some couples do embark on separation as a trial period of, say, from three to six months to see how they do on their own and to see what becomes of their relationship in the interim. Some of these couples separate taking it a week at a time, with a loose arrangement about when and how much they see each other, whether they date others, and so forth. Some elect at the outset not to see each other (except for the children, when there are children), to keep their lives as separate and as private as possible, and to meet at the end of an agreed-upon time interval to see how they feel about each other and whether they wish to attempt and work toward a reconciliation. Still other couples separate when one or both feel very ambivalent about their relationship; that is, the relationship does not seem completely over, but it has gone beyond the trial separation stage. They suspect that the separation will be permanent but they are not sure. Finally, other couples separate knowing they will divorce. These couples are in the minority.

One question I am asked repeatedly by individuals whose spouses would like a trial separation that they do not agree with is, "Isn't a trial separation just a euphemism, a nice term, a gentle term for divorce?" It isn't really. People wanting a trial separation are not 100% clear—they usually want some distance and independence from their spouse, but they are never certain that they want a divorce at that point. Although many couples who attempt a trial separation do not get back together and go on to divorce eventually, there are many others who reconcile and remain together happily. Indeed, there are many couples in our society who state quite boldly, and proudly, that they would not be together today had they not separated temporarily at an earlier time in their marriage. The question about trial separation being a euphemism comes from a position of vulnerability, of feeling rejected, unloved, hurt, angry, and frightened. These feelings are summed up in the statement,

"Don't beat around the bush with me. Hit me over the head with it. Say it. You don't love me anymore. Let's just get on with it—divorce me!"

As you can see, your therapist can assist the two of you in talking about these separation options and their accompanying dynamics. They are not easy to talk about. Even if you and your spouse are able to discuss them calmly and rationally, there may be something much more tumultuous going on inside each of you. You may wish to meet individually with your therapist for several sessions after separating, because your needs will be different and there will be things to talk about that are not appropriate to a conjoint format. Your therapist may wish to meet with you together from time to time if there are concerns about the children or if there are disagreements and hurt feelings about how much time you spend together. One of you may feel quite private about your living space and feel that your spouse does not respect or understand that. One of you may not wish to see the other alone except to discuss the children, whereas your spouse would like to "date" you. One of you may wish to get together occasionally as a family but the other disagrees, feeling that meeting that way would confuse the children. One of you may have concerns about the other's "morals," especially regarding sleeping arrangements when having a new man or woman friend stay overnight while the children are present. These are a few of the many issues that are more easily discussed and resolved with a therapist's help.

WHAT ABOUT INDIVIDUAL TREATMENT?

Earlier in this chapter, I talked about individual treatment being suggested by your therapist for yourself or your spouse or both of you. I emphasized the importance of your having a clear and acceptable rationale from your therapist about the recommendation of individual therapy. Only in this way can you begin to feel less focused on or singled out. Then, in therapy, you can approach your difficulties with less trepidation and less defensiveness. I want now to talk about the benefits and improved feelings about one's self that can accrue from individual therapy.

It seems to me that the long-standing tradition of women requesting and accepting psychiatric help more readily than men continues. More men are coming forward than in the past, and they come earlier, but there is still a gender gap. Within medicine, it is more common for distressed medical students, residents, and younger physicians to request psychiatric help than it is for older physicians. But here there is a gender gap, too. In my practice, I find that it is more common that the initial call for marital help comes from the woman in the relationship, regardless of whether or not she is a medical student or physician. When a male doctor does call me about a marital problem and requests marital therapy, he is often designated to make the call at his wife's insistence because things are terrible and she can't stand it anymore. Or a male doctor may call wanting his wife to come in with him for marital work after it is too late; she has already decided to leave and doesn't want any professional help at all or wants separation therapy.

I think that seeing a therapist for marital problems is easier, less threatening, and more acceptable than going for individual therapy. I know that many of my patients, physicians included, prefer to see me as a marital therapist, *not* a psychiatrist. It's OK to have marital problems; it's not OK to have personal problems. "We're seeing a marriage counselor" sounds better than "We're seeing a psychiatrist about our marriage." I am also aware of how surprised some doctors and their spouses are if, in the course of this conjoint work with me, one of them becomes quite symptomatic and requires medication, or even hospitalization. "Forgive me, but I had forgotten that you're a doctor, aren't you?" sums up the feeling.

I have seen countless couples over the years whose marital problem was the "ticket" to individual therapy for one or both of them. Confronting marital tension and unhappiness is the first time that many individuals are forced to take a hard, cold look at themselves, and this can be sobering. Personal weaknesses and fears, often identified by one's spouse, stand out in bold relief. Even if you've been conscious of them earlier in life, it was easier then to bury them, to shrug them off, or (and this is common in medical students and doctors) to sublimate them into something noble such as study or work. "I thought of seeing a psychiatrist when I was in medical school (or residency) but just kept putting it off" is a not uncommon response made by maritally distressed doctors to my suggestion about doing some individual therapy with them. Most welcome the opportunity and work eagerly and creatively at it.

There are some common themes that characterize what doctors work on in individual therapy: unresolved grief from earlier losses in their lives, especially the death of a parent or sibling and, increasingly in young doctors, their parents' divorce; conflicts about medicine as a career choice and life's work, in particular disillusionment and lack of personal satisfaction (this can be quite marked in doctors coming from families with lengthy medical lineage); underlying problems with self-esteem and self-confidence, especially in social and sexual matters, hiding behind a professional image of competence and success; conflicts with intimacy both in marriage and in friendship despite being quite sociable, popular, and well liked by others; reconciling career with one's personal and family life (a special problem for women doctors, but becoming more so for men); loneliness and personal isolation outside of medicine (this seems to be more common in male doctors who depend too heavily on their wives to counteract this feeling or keep it out of conscious awareness).[10]

Some physicians never consider individual therapy until after their marriages have ended, even though they may have had personal or marital problems before. There are many reasons for coming, but one of the most common is a sense that they are not progressing as quickly as they feel they should be. Here is an example:[11]

Tony was a thirty-three-year-old emergency room physician who came to see me eight months after he and his wife separated. He began the visit with the following statement: "I feel rather foolish being here. . . . I can't seem to get it together about being separated. . . . I can't seem to get on with my life. . . . I'm the one who left the marriage, and I'm relieved to be on my own. . . . I just can't figure out why I'm not happier." Tony went on to tell me that he felt physically very well, that he was doing his work with no difficulty, and that he exercised on a regular basis. He was going out with a woman whom he described in very positive terms and whom he planned to continue to see. He denied feeling depressed, and indeed he certainly didn't look or sound very depressed. He had spoken to one of his male friends about the way he was feeling, but that was not very helpful—he came away feeling he had just made a fool of himself.

On more careful examination, there were two findings that concerned me about Tony. First, he was awakening very early in the morning, about four a.m., and he was unable to return to sleep. Being quite driven, he didn't think too much of this; he decided to use the extra hours of wakefulness to work on a sailboat that he was building. Second, when I asked him if he had ever had any psychiatric troubles in the past, he said no. However, a bit later in the interview he told me that he had had two periods of complete emotional and social withdrawal as a medical student. The first was in his second year of medical school, and it lasted two weeks. He took the phone off the hook, didn't go outdoors, and lost about ten pounds because he wasn't eating. He suddenly felt better and returned to classes. The second episode was similar, except this time he felt severely depressed; he had a well-organized plan to hang himself from a rafter in his basement apartment if he did not feel better by a certain date. Fortunately, he spontaneously began to feel well again.

I made a provisional diagnosis of clinical depression and kept a close eye on Tony's mood throughout the course of our work together. He responded very well to supportive psychotherapy and did not require medication.

With many medical couples I use an integrated model of therapy that combines conjoint and individual treatment. Weeks of conjoint work may be followed by a course of individual treatment, followed by conjoint work again in an alternating pattern, as necessary. There is a dynamic interplay between the two approaches. The conjoint visits serve to identify the areas of conflict and allow some resolution; the individual work allows the exposition, the uncovering, and the working through of the rest. I have found that the more intensive one-on-one psychotherapy is not possible without the earlier conjoint work, and the later conjoint work cannot proceed without the intervening individual work. This is what I meant earlier about marital distress becoming the ticket to individual work.

If you or your spouse are reluctant to seek or start with individual therapy, conjoint work is beneficial. It not only helps settle the problems but gives you an opportunity to establish some rapport with your therapist. To be frank, you get a chance to observe, to assess, to come to "know" him or her as the interaction between your therapist and each of you unfolds. You can determine how comfortable, trusting, or interested you are in individual treatment. Male doctors and husbands of women doctors who have gone on to do some individual therapy with me have often commented how their initial cynicism and disparaging attitude toward psychotherapy had been alleviated by this "soft sell" introduction.

I would like to conclude this chapter by quoting an orthopedic surgeon patient of mine, whom I saw both with his wife and alone, as he summed up his work with me in his final session: "When I was a medical student, if someone had told me that fifteen years down the road I'd be seeing a psychiatrist, I would've decked him. Not for assuming I'd have problems, but that I'd take them to a shrink! I've never had any understanding of what you guys do, and I still don't understand it, but something has happened to me in coming here that I can't describe. I know that you know that it wasn't easy for me to come here, but you really don't know how hard it was—nobody knows. But I can tell you that approaching death will be a hell of a lot easier for me than it was to come here! I am changed in some way. I know I'm a happier man, at peace in some way. It's hard to put my finger on it. My wife says I'm a different person, but she's always been prone to hyperbole. My kids . . .

well *(he becomes tearful).* I think it's time to go now and let you get on with your next patient."

REFERENCES

1. Michael F. Myers, "Marital Distress Among Resident Physicians," *Canadian Medical Association Journal* 134 (May 15, 1986), 1117–1118.
2. William J. Doherty, Mary Ellen Lester, and Geoffrey Leigh, "Marriage Encounter Weekends: Couples Who Win and Couples Who Lose," *Journal of Marital and Family Therapy* 12 (January 1986), 49–61.
3. Alan S. Gurman, "The Effects and Effectiveness of Marital Therapy," in *Couples in Conflict,* ed. Alan S. Gurman and David G. Rice (New York: Jason Aronson, 1975), 383–406.
4. Neil S. Jacobson, "A Review of the Research on the Effectiveness of Marital Therapy," in *Marriage and Marital Therapy: Psychoanalytic, Behavioral, and Systems Theory Perspectives,* ed. Thomas J. Paolino and Barbara S. McCrady (New York: Brunner/Mazel, 1978), 395–444.
5. Michael F. Myers, "Treating Troubled Marriages," *American Family Physician* 29 (January 1984), 221–226.
6. Fitzhugh Mullan, Robert M. Politzer, Caroline T. Lewis, Stanford Bastacky, John Rodak, and Robert G. Harmon, "The National Practitioner Data Bank: Report from the First Year," *Journal of the American Medical Association* 268 (July 1, 1992), 73–79.
7. Kathleen M. Mogul, "Overview: The Sex of the Therapist," *American Journal of Psychiatry* 139 (January 1982), 1–11.
8. Michael F. Myers, "Fighting Stigma: How to Help the Doctor's Family," in *Stigma and Mental Illness,* ed. P. J. Fink and A. Tasman (Washington, D.C.: American Psychiatric Press, 1992), 139–150.
9. Michael F. Myers, "Types of Marital Therapy in Psychiatric Practice," in *Marital Therapy in Psychiatric Practice,* ed. E. Waring and L. Frelick (New York: Brunner/Mazel, 1987), 80–103.
10. Michael F. Myers, "Treating Physicians with Psychotherapy," *Directions in Psychiatry,* 12 (June 26, 1992), 1–8.
11. Michael F. Myers, *Men and Divorce* (New York: Guilford, 1989), 218.

INDEX

Gay-bashing, 108–109, 183
Gay males, 110–118. *See also* Sexual orienta-
    tion conflicts
    age discrepancy in, 114–116
    AIDS and, 107, 108, 111, 117–118, 127,
        183, 195
    coming-out and, 113–114, 126
    competition between, 110–111
    as fathers, 116–117
    intimacy problems in, 113
    issues specific for physicians, 124–128
    parents of, 109, 181–184
    sexual acting out in, 111–112
    social prejudice against, 108–110
Gay marriages, 108
Geographical relocation, 7–10
Gestalt theory, 232
Gilligan, Carol, 82, 93, 119
Grief, 8, 180
Group therapy, 233
Guilt
    alleviation of, 213–214
    female physicians and, 78–79

Hashish, 58
Here-and-now techniques, 232
Homophobia, 108, 109, 120, 123
Homosexuals. *See* Gay males; Lesbians
Husbands
    fear of abandonment in, 39
    illness in, 175
    of medical students, 2, 24–26
    of resident physicians, 2, 4
    under- or unemployed, 96–97
    with unmet needs, 85–87
    who feel belittled, 90–91
Hyperactivity, 176–177
Hypomania, 191

Illnesses, 163–164, 171–176. *See also* Psychi-
    atric illnesses
Impostor phenomenon, 97–98
*In a Different Voice: Psychological Theory
    and Women's Development* (Gilligan), 82
Incest, 12, 121, 236–237. *See also* Sexual
    abuse
Individual therapy, 233–235, 246–250
Intermarriage, 30–32, 196–198
International Doctors in AA (IDAA),
    70, 104

International medical graduates (IMG),
    41–42, 196–198
Intimacy problems
    in female physicians, 87–88
    in gay males, 113
Intravenous drug abuse, 194–195

Jewish physicians, 217
Joint custody, 142, 147

Lawsuits. *See* Malpractice suits
Learning disabilities, 176–177
Lesbians, 111, 118–124
    coming-out of, 119–121, 126
    conflicts of closeness and distance in,
        118–119
    issues specific for physicians and,
        124–128
    as mothers, 122–124
    parents of, 109, 181–184
    separation problems in, 123–124
    sexual problems and, 121
    social prejudice against, 108–110
Life Stress Events Scale, 131
Lithium, 192
Loneliness/isolation, 7–10, 28
Loss, 160–162, 164
*Love and Tradition: Marriage between Jews
    and Christians* (Mayer), 31
Lubrication difficulties, 63

Male physicians, 47–72
    alcoholism in, 56–57
    communication problems and, 48–54
    depression in, 58–62
    divorce and, 133–139, 150
    overwork in, 54–56
    self-medication in, 57–58
    sexual problems and, 62–69
Male resident physicians, 3–4, 40
Malpractice suits, 189–191, 218
Mania, 163
Manic–depressive illness, 62, 177–178, 185,
    192, 242
Marijuana, 58
Marital enrichment programs, 208–209
Marital rape, 101, 121
Marital therapy, 201–251
    benefits of, 211–214
    delay in seeking, 75–78